ANATOMY, PHYSIOLOGY, AND PATHOLOGY WORKBOOK

Study Tools, Practices, and Exercises for Students to Understand the Human Body

Third Edition

Ruth Hull

lotus
publishing

Chichester, England

North Atlantic Books

Huichin, unceded Ohlone land
Berkeley, California

This third edition published in 2024 by
Lotus Publishing
Apple Tree Cottage, Inlands Road, Nutbourne, Chichester, PO18 8RJ, and
North Atlantic Books
Huichin, unceded Ohlone land
Berkeley, California

Text Design Medlar Publishing Solutions Pvt Ltd., India
Cover Design Chris Fulcher
Printed and Bound Kultur Sanat Printing House, Turkey

Anatomy, Physiology, and Pathology Workbook, Third Edition: Study Tools, Practices, and Exercises for Students to Understand the Human Body is sponsored and published by North Atlantic Books, an educational nonprofit based on the unceded Ohlone land Huichin (Berkeley, CA), that collaborates with partners to develop cross-cultural perspectives, nurture holistic views of art, science, the humanities, and healing, and seed personal and global transformation by publishing work on the relationship of body, spirit, and nature.

North Atlantic Books's publications are distributed to the US trade and internationally by Penguin Random House Publishers Services. For further information, visit our website at www.northatlanticbooks.com.

MEDICAL DISCLAIMER: The following information is intended for general information purposes only. Individuals should always see their healthcare provider before administering any suggestions made in this book. Any application of the material set forth in the following pages is at the reader's discretion and is their sole responsibility.

British Library Cataloguing-in-Publication Data
A CIP record for this book is available from the British Library
ISBN 978 1 913088 41 5 (Lotus Publishing)
ISBN 979 8 88984 124 1 (North Atlantic Books)

Library of Congress Cataloging-in-Publication Data
Names: Hull, Ruth, author.
Title: Anatomy, physiology, and pathology workbook, third edition :
    study tools, practices, and exercises for students to understand
    the human body / Ruth Hull.
Description: Third edition. | Chichester, England ; Berkeley, California :
    Lotus Publications, North Atlantic Book, 2024.
Identifiers: LCCN 2024000975 (print) | LCCN 2024000976 (ebook) |
    ISBN 9798889841241 (trade paperback) | ISBN 9798889841258 (ebook)
Subjects: LCSH: Anatomy | MESH: Physiological Phenomena |
    Pathologic Processes | Signs and Symptoms
Classification: LCC QP34.5 .H84 2024 (print) | LCC QP34.5 (ebook) |
    DDC 612--dc23/eng/20240130
LC record available at https://lccn.loc.gov/2024000975
LC ebook record available at https://lccn.loc.gov/2024000976

Contents

A Note on American and British Spellings

This book uses US spelling conventions, and some of the technical ones may be unfamiliar to students from the UK or elsewhere. A list of these is provided below. Students should be aware of these different spellings as they may encounter them in their future studies or work.

The list doesn't include examples of the simple s/z difference, such as in "mineralised" and "catalysed" (UK) versus "mineralized" and "catalyzed" (US). And some of the more common words—e.g., the American "millimeter," "gray," and "odor" versus the British "millimetre," "grey," and "odour"—are likewise not included here.

For the most part, the differences in spelling are minor; for example, "ae" in the British "anaemia" and "haemoglobin" versus just "e" in the US "anemia" and "hemoglobin." Or "oe" in the British "oestrogen" and "oesophagus" versus just "e" in the American "estrogen" and "esophagus."

There is an exception, however, where the most common term in the US is an entirely different word to the one most commonly used in the UK: "epinephrine" is the preferred American form for what the British mostly call "adrenaline." The same difference is seen with "norepinephrine" and "noradrenaline." This book uses "epinephrine" and "norepinephrine," but in places readers will see "adrenaline" and "noradrenaline" also, as a reminder.

BRITISH/AMERICAN SPELLING DIFFERENCES OF TECHNICAL TERMS

British term	US term
adrenaline	epinephrine
aetiology	etiology
aluminium	aluminum
amenorrhoea	amenorrhea
anaemia	anemia
anaesthetise	anesthetize
bacteraemia	bacteremia
caecum	cecum
coeliac	celiac
diarrhoea	diarrhea
dyslipidaemia	dyslipidemia
dysmenorrhoea	dysmenorrhea

BRITISH/AMERICAN SPELLING DIFFERENCES OF TECHNICAL TERMS

British term	US term
dyspnoea	dyspnea
faeces	feces
foetus, foetal	fetus, fetal
galactorrhoea	galactorrhea
goitre	goiter
gonorrhoea	gonorrhea
gynaecologist	gynecologist
gynaecomastia	gynecomastia
haematoma	hematoma
haematuria	hematuria
haemoglobin	hemoglobin
haemophilia	hemophilia
haemopoiesis	hemopoiesis
haemoptysis	hemoptysis
haemorrhage, haemorrhagic	hemorrhage, hemorrhagic
haemorrhoids	hemorrhoids
haemostasis	hemostasis
humour	humor
hypercholesterolaemia	hypercholesterolemia
hyperglycaemia	hyperglycemia
hypertriglyceridaemia	hypertriglyceridemia
hypocalcaemia	hypocalcemia
hypoglycaemia	hypoglycemia
ileocaecal	ileocecal
ischaemia, ischaemic	ischemia, ischemic
leukaemia	leukemia
lymphoedema	lymphedema
mould	mold
myxoedema	myxedema
noradrenaline	norepinephrine
oedema	edema
oesophageal	esophageal
oesophagitis	esophagitis
oesophagus	esophagus
oestradiol	estradiol
oestriol	estriol
oestrogen, oestrogenic	estrogen, estrogenic
oestrone	estrone
onychogryphosis	onychogryposis
oxyhaemoglobin	oxyhemoglobin
seborrhoea	seborrhea
septicaemia	septicemia
sulphur	sulfur
thalassaemia	thalassemia
tumour	tumor

PART 1

Introduction

Welcome to our anatomy, physiology, and pathology workbook. The purpose of this book is to help you succeed in the difficult task of learning the anatomy and physiology of the human body. To do this, it has been written in three parts.

Part 1

First, the body has been broken down into systems, and each system is represented by a chapter in which:

- You are first guided through making your own review and self-study notes. This section suggests exercises that will help you to both understand and learn the facts you need to know. You may come across some study tips or suggestions for group work. **Please note, answers are not provided for this section.**
- You then work through a series of questions and exercises that will test your knowledge of the body system you are studying. These questions include a section on the pathology of the system, a short vocabulary test, and multiple-choice questions. **Answers to all these exercises are provided at the end of the book.**

Part 2

Once you have covered all the chapters in part 1 and you feel confident that you have a sound understanding of each system and a good knowledge of the facts, you can move on to part 2 of the workbook. This section is made up of 14 practice quizzes, each one covering the entire anatomy and physiology syllabus. Pretend you are taking an exam and, under exam conditions, work through a practice quiz. When you mark it, make a note of the questions you got wrong and your weak areas. Before moving on to the next multiple-choice quiz, spend some time reviewing your weak areas.

Part 3

In the final part of this workbook it is your turn to bring all your learning together, to deepen your understanding of both health and disease and to put your knowledge into action.

Memory Techniques

Some of the review and study-guide exercises ask you to draw mind maps or spider diagrams, write flash cards, or create mnemonics. This is how to do it. **Remember—nobody else needs to see any of these so don't worry if you are not an artist!**

Mind maps and spider diagrams

Mind maps are simple diagrams that help you link thoughts, ideas, or information. They are fun to create, and it is while creating them that you begin to understand and enjoy what you are learning. It is also easier to remember images that you have personally created than to remember text that has been written by somebody else.

How to create a mind map:

- Take the text that you need to learn or understand and underline the key ideas. Now convert these written ideas into images.
- On a blank piece of paper draw the central idea and, surrounding it, draw the other ideas.
- Link them up with arrows or lines.

What is important when creating a map is to use words, colors, pictures, or symbols that are personal to YOU. Use things that you will remember.

A practical example of a mind map

This example has been taken from chapter 3 where you need to learn about eccrine glands. The "e" is for eccrine, the hands and feet are reminders of the location, the thermometer is a reminder of their function, and the sweaty face is a reminder of their excretion.

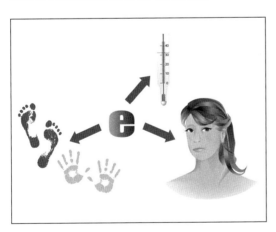

Flash cards and sticky notes

Flash cards and sticky notes are short, simple review notes that contain only the facts that need to be memorized. When you create and use flash cards, remember to:

- Write important definitions, names, dates, etc., on little cards that you can carry with you everywhere you go. When stuck in a line or waiting for a bus you can have a quick look at one or two of them.
- Write important points on sticky notes and stick them on your refrigerator, bathroom door, telephone, bathroom mirror, or anything you see on a daily basis.
- The important thing is to keep them short and simple. Use color and/or symbols.

A practical example of a flash card

The word "caudal" means away from the head or below.

Caudal

Front of card

Away from the head, below.

Back of card

Mnemonics

Mnemonics are words, sentences, or verses created to help you remember information. When you create a mnemonic, remember to:

- Write a list of the facts you need to recall.
- Underline the first letter of each fact.
- Create a rhyme, phrase, or word that you will easily remember using these letters.

The more personal, fun, and amusing these phrases are, the more easily you will remember them.

Practical example of a mnemonic

The epidermis of the skin is composed of five layers. These are the strata:

• Basale
• Spinosum
• Granulosum
• Lucidum
• Corneum

Mnemonic: Bad skin grafts look comical.

Tips for the Coloring-in Exercises

When completing the coloring-in exercises, be sure to do it slowly and mindfully as this is your chance to really integrate your learning.

• Always start with the key and work with one structure at a time. Write the function or description of the structure into the key and choose a color for that structure.
• Then slowly color the structure you have chosen, and as you color it repeat to yourself its name and function.

Work slowly through this book and enjoy it. Remember, you learn best when you are having fun.

We didn't realize we were making memories, we just knew we were having fun.

—Winnie the Pooh

---

1 Before You Begin

Review/Self–Study Notes

Before you can study anatomy you need to have a good knowledge of anatomical terminology. Unfortunately, the only way to learn this terminology is by memorizing it. To help you do this, make flash cards of the following terms and their definitions.

Anatomy	Ventral	Pelvic	Patellar
Physiology	Cutaneous	Inguinal	Popliteal
Pathology	Cephalic	Pubic	Sural
Anatomical position	Facial	Perineal	Tarsal
Anterior	Frontal	Acromial	Pedal
Posterior	Ophthalmic/orbital	Scapular	Calcaneal
Dorsal	Otic	Axillary	Plantar
Superior	Buccal	Brachial	Parietal
Inferior	Nasal	Cubital	Visceral
Medial	Occipital	Antecubital	Sagittal plane
Lateral	Cervical	Olecranal	Frontal/coronal
Proximal	Thoracic	Antebrachial	plane
Distal	Costal	Carpal	Transverse plane/
Superficial	Pericardial	Manual	cross-section
Deep	Mammary	Palmar/metacarpal	Oblique plane
Peripheral	Abdominal	Digital/phalangeal	Quadrant
Cephalad	Umbilical	Gluteal	Cavity
Cranial	Lumbar	Crural	
Caudal	Coxal	Femoral	

Study tip

Write the definitions in your own words. It is always easier to remember your own words than someone else's.

Study groups

To help you revise your terminology, play the game "30 seconds." Here's how to do it:

30 seconds

Preparation:
1. Make or buy some small cards. On each card write down five different anatomical terms. The more cards you have, the longer the game will be.
2. Get a clock or stopwatch so that you will be able to time 30 seconds per round.
3. Divide yourselves into two teams (teams A and B).

To play:
1. One member from team A will stand up, take a card, and quickly read the five terms silently.
2. That person then has to describe each term to the other members of team A without saying the term written on the card.
3. The teammates need to guess and call out the terms written on the card. They will get one point for each term they identify correctly.
4. Each team has only 30 seconds in which to go through the terms on the card.
5. At the end of the round, write down how many points that team has obtained.
6. It is then team B's turn.
7. At the end of the game, when all the cards have been used up, add up the points each team has gained. The team with the most points wins!

Exercises

1. This figure shows a man standing in the anatomical position. Label the arrows with the directional terms listed on the right.

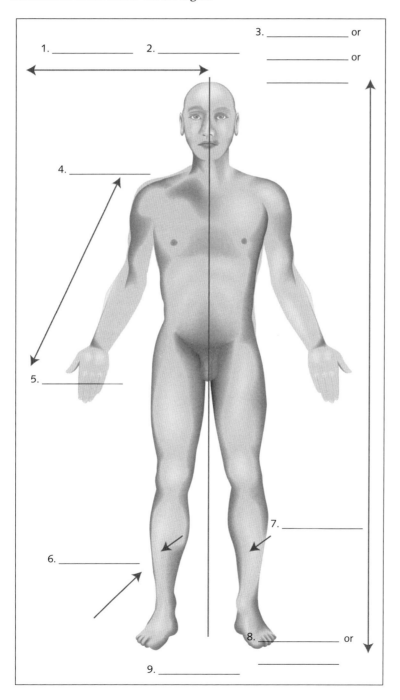

3. _____ or

_____ or

_____

1. _____   2. _____

4. _____

5. _____

6. _____

7. _____

8. _____ or

_____

9. _____

| Median line |
| Superior |
| Inferior |
| Medial |
| Lateral |
| Proximal |
| Distal |
| Superficial |
| Deep |
| Cephalad |
| Cranial |
| Caudal |

2. **Using directional terms, fill in the blanks.**

   a. The heart is _____ to the stomach.

   b. The diaphragm is _____ to the lungs.

   c. The heart is _____ to the lungs.

   d. The lungs are _____ to the heart.

   e. The knee is _____ to the ankle.

   f. The ankle is _____ to the knee.

   g. The hands and feet are at the _____ of the body.

3. **Match the anatomical term to the region it describes.**

Anatomical term:	Region described:
1. Buccal	a. Hollow behind the knee
2. Cephalic	
3. Dorsal	b. Back
4. Phalangeal	c. Elbow or forearm
5. Cubital	d. Head
6. Inguinal	e. Heart
7. Popliteal	f. Skin
8. Pericardial	g. Fingers or toes
9. Sural	h. Cheek
10. Cutaneous	i. Calf
	j. Groin

   Answers:

   1. _____ 2. _____ 3. _____ 4. _____

   5. _____ 6. _____ 7. _____ 8. _____

   9. _____ 10. _____

4. **The figure below shows the cavities of the body. Label the cavities and place the organs listed into the cavities in which they belong.**

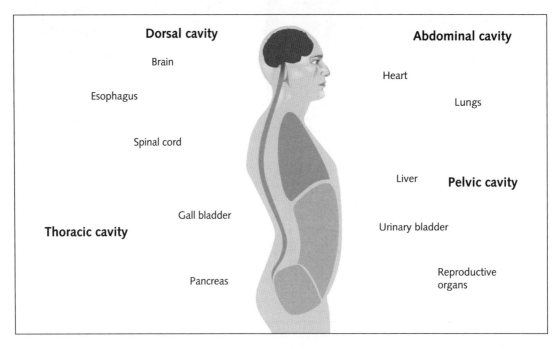

Dorsal cavity

Brain

Esophagus

Spinal cord

Gall bladder

Thoracic cavity

Pancreas

Abdominal cavity

Heart

Lungs

Liver   **Pelvic cavity**

Urinary bladder

Reproductive organs

5. The figure below shows the planes of the body. Label them.

a. _____   b. _____   c. _____   d. _____

6. Are the following conditions acute or chronic?

    a. Emphysema _____

    b. Hyperventilation _____

    c. Asthmatic attack _____

    d. Influenza _____

    e. Diabetes mellitus _____

    f. Varicose veins _____

    g. Fibromyalgia _____

    h. Ankle sprain _____

    i. Syncope _____

    j. Pharyngitis _____

7. Are the following conditions systemic or localized?

    a. Sinusitis _____

    b. Ankle sprain _____

    c. Tennis elbow _____

    d. AIDS _____

    e. Seasonal affective disorder (SAD) _____

    f. Cushing's syndrome _____

    g. Rhinitis _____

    h. Anemia _____

    i. Constipation _____

    j. Cataract _____

8. Are the following signs or symptoms?

    a. Yellowing of the skin _____

    b. Hearing loss _____

    c. Tingling sensation _____

    d. Fever _____

    e. Perspiration _____

    f. Nausea _____

    g. Vomiting _____

    h. Diarrhea _____

    i. Headache _____

    j. Fatigue _____

9. **Thinking about the effects of stress on the body, fill in the blanks.**

   When put under short-term stress such as being physically threatened, our (a) _____ nervous system responds with a (b) "_____ -or- _____ response." Hormones secreted as part of this response are (c) _____ and norepinephrine (noradrenaline). Long-term stress, such as the death of a loved one, involves different hormones. The most significant hormone in long-term stress is (d) _____.

Vocabulary test

Complete the table below.

WORD	DEFINITION
Anatomy	a. _____
Cephalad	b. _____
Cross-section	c. _____
Distal	d. _____
Midline	e. _____
Parietal	f. _____
Pathology	g. _____
Physiology	h. _____
Ventral	i. _____
Visceral	j. _____
k. _____	Diseases that begin suddenly and are short-lived and resolvable
l. _____	Muscle wasting
m. _____	The excessive accumulation of interstitial fluid in body tissues
n. _____	The doctor's opinion of how a disease will progress and what will be the most likely outcome for the patient
o. _____	A common immune response to injury or invasion, characterized by swelling, warmth, redness, pain, and sometimes loss of movement

WORD	DEFINITION
p. _____	Term indicating "at the surface or outer part of the body"
q. _____	Anatomical term for the wrist
r. _____	Term to describe diseases that are ongoing, persistent, and not always resolvable
s. _____	Term used to describe a condition that involves the entire body
t. _____	Term used to describe the cause or origin of a disease

Multiple-Choice Questions

1. Which of the following phrases is correct?
   a. Anatomy is the study of the functions of the body
   b. Anatomy is the study of the diseases of the body
   c. Anatomy is the study of the structure of the body
   d. Anatomy is the study of the pathology of the body

2. If a man is standing in the anatomical position he will be standing:
   a. Facing forward with his arms hanging by his sides and his palms facing forward
   b. Facing forward with his arms hanging by his sides and his palms facing backward
   c. Facing backward with his arms hanging by his sides and his palms facing forward
   d. Facing backward with his arms hanging by his sides and his palms facing backward

3. Another term for the midline is:
   a. The middle line
   b. The median line
   c. The medial line
   d. The periphery

4. Which of the following phrases is correct?
   a. The term "cephalad" means toward the feet
   b. The term "deep" means toward the surface of the body
   c. The term "proximal" means further from the point of attachment of a limb
   d. The term "dorsal" means at the back of the body

5. Which of the following structures are all located in the abdominal cavity?
   a. Stomach, urinary bladder, reproductive organs
   b. Liver, spleen, gall bladder
   c. Pancreas, small intestine, bronchi
   d. Lungs, heart, diaphragm

6. The term "calcaneal" describes which region of the body?
   a. Thigh
   b. Calf
   c. Ankle
   d. Heel

7. What is the anatomical term used to describe the hips?
   a. Coxal
   b. Inguinal
   c. Costal
   d. Umbilical

8. The term "parietal" relates to:
   a. The internal organs of the body
   b. The external organs of the body
   c. The inner walls of a body cavity
   d. The external walls of a body cavity

9. What type of plane divides the body vertically into posterior and anterior portions?
   a. Coronal
   b. Transverse
   c. Sagittal
   d. Oblique

10. What is the collective name of the regions that the abdominopelvic cavity can be divided into?
    a. Fifths
    b. Quadrants
    c. Quarters
    d. Thirds

2 Organization of the Body

Review/Self–Study Notes

Levels of structural and chemical organization of the body

When you first start studying anatomy it helps to have a basic understanding of how the body is organized and the chemicals it is made up of.

1. List the six levels of structural organization of the body.

   * _____

   * _____

   * _____

   * _____

   * _____

   * _____

2. Name the four major elements that make up 96% of the body's mass.

   * _____

   * _____

   * _____

   * _____

3. Create a mnemonic (see "Mnemonics" section of the introduction) for the nine lesser elements in the body. These are:
   * Calcium
   * Phosphorus
   * Potassium
   * Sulfur
   * Sodium
   * Chlorine
   * Magnesium

   * Iodine
   * Iron

   Mnemonic: _____

   _____

4. Describe each of the following compounds and its role in the body.

   a. Water _____

   _____

   _____

   b. Carbohydrates _____

   _____

   _____

   _____

   c. Lipids (fats) _____

   _____

   _____

   _____

   d. Proteins _____

   _____

   _____

   _____

e. Nucleic acids _____   f. Adenosine triphosphate _____

_____   _____

_____   _____

_____

Cellular organization of the body

Cells are the basic structural and functional units of the body and although there are many different types of cell, they generally have the same basic makeup. They are surrounded by a plasma membrane, which regulates the movement of all substances into and out of the cell.

5. Describe the structure and function of the plasma membrane in your own words.

_____

_____

6. Below is a simplified plasma membrane. Take your time to color in and label the image. Remember to work with one structure at a time. Start by writing the function/description of the structure and coloring in the "color" box in the key. Then color in that structure on the image and repeat the name and function to yourself as you color in.

KEY: PLASMA MEMBRANE		
Structure	**Function/Description**	**Color**
Phospholipid bilayer		This only needs to be labeled; it does not need to be colored
Phospholipid head		
Phospholipid tail		
Integral protein		
Peripheral protein		
Cholesterol		

7. Substances can be transported across the plasma membrane by a number of different processes. Describe each of the following processes in no more than ten words. The first one has been done for you.

   a. Simple diffusion <u>from high</u>

      <u>concentration to low concentration</u>

   b. Osmosis _____

      _____

   c. Facilitated diffusion _____

      _____

   d. Active transport _____

      _____

   e. Vesicular transport _____

      _____

8. Imagine the cell is a factory, and list all the cell structures as parts of that factory. A similar example to this is given in chapter 2 of *Anatomy, Physiology, and Pathology* (Hull, 2023), where the cell has been likened to a bakery (e.g., the plasma membrane is the walls and doors of the building).

   The cell as a factory:

   - Plasma membrane _____
   - Cytoplasm _____
   - Nucleus _____
   - Mitochondria _____
   - Ribosomes _____
   - Endoplasmic reticulum _____
   - Golgi complex _____
   - Lysosomes _____
   - Peroxisomes _____

9. In the box below, draw a spider diagram or mind map showing the life cycle of a cell.

Now color in the cell below. Remember to start by completing the key first.

KEY: GENERALIZED CELL		
Structure	Function/Description	Color
Cell membrane		
Cytoplasm		
Nuclear envelope		

KEY: GENERALIZED CELL		
Structure	Function/Description	Color
Rough endoplasmic reticulum		
Chromatin		
Centriole		
Smooth endoplasmic reticulum		
Glycogen		
Nucleus		
Nucleolus		
Microtubules		
Mitochondrion		
Lysosome		
Vacuole		
Golgi apparatus		
Ribosomes		
Microvilli		
Microfilament		

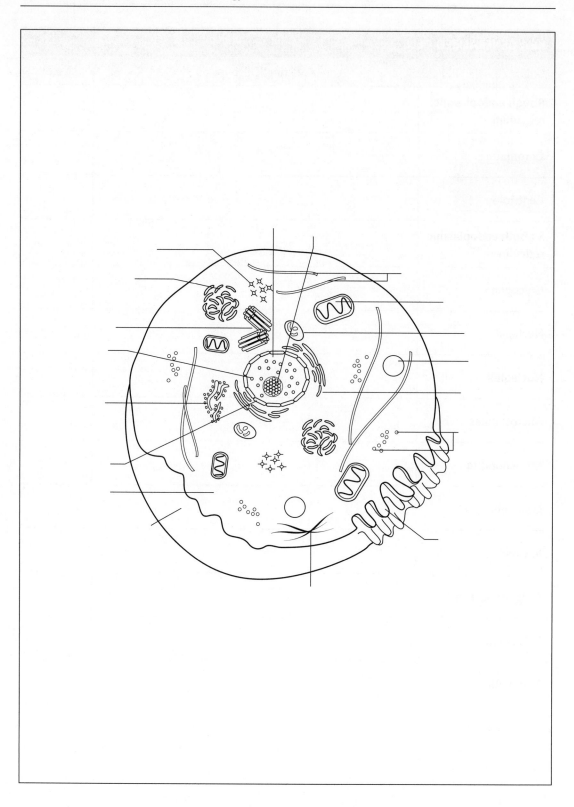

Tissue level of organization of the body

Tissues are composed of groups of similar cells all working together to perform a common function.

10. Complete the following table on tissues in the body. The first key phrase has been done for you.

TYPES OF TISSUE IN THE BODY			
Name	Description	Function	Example
Epithelial			
Key phrase to remember: Epithelial tissue covers and lines.			
Connective			
Key phrase to remember:			
Muscle			
Key phrase to remember:			
Nervous			
Key phrase to remember:			

11. There are so many different types of tissue in the body that it is often difficult to remember them all. For each tissue listed below write down no more than five words that will remind you of it. The first one has been done for you.
Epithelial tissue:

- Simple squamous (pavement) epithelium single, flat, lining _____
- Simple cuboidal epithelium _____
- Simple columnar epithelium _____
- Ciliated simple columnar epithelium _____
- Stratified squamous epithelium _____
- Transitional epithelium _____

In order to remind yourself of epithelial classification, remember that there are different cell **shapes** (types) that make up epithelial tissue. Color and label these below.

KEY: TYPES OF EPITHELIAL TISSUE CELLS	
Type/Shape	**Color**
Columnar	
Squamous	
Cuboidal	
Ciliated	
Transitional	Note: This shape has not been included as it looks the same as columnar

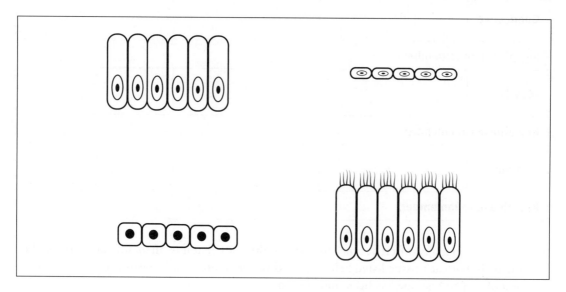

Connective tissue:

- Areolar tissue _____
- Adipose tissue _____
- Lymphoid (reticular) tissue _____
- Elastic connective (yellow elastic) tissue _____
- Dense regular connective (white fibrous) tissue _____
- Osseous tissue (bone) _____

- Hyaline cartilage _____
- Fibrocartilage _____
- Elastic cartilage _____
- Vascular tissue (blood) _____

Muscle tissue:

- Skeletal muscle tissue _____
- Cardiac muscle tissue _____
- Smooth (visceral) muscle tissue _____

Nervous tissue:

- _____

_____

_____

Membranes:

- Mucous membranes _____

_____

_____

- Serous membranes _____

_____

_____

- Connective tissue (synovial) membranes _____

_____

_____

The diagrams below illustrate the different types of muscle tissue: skeletal, cardiac, and smooth. It is quite easy to tell which is smooth muscle tissue, but more difficult to tell the difference between skeletal and cardiac muscle tissues. To help you differentiate, complete the following table and then color in and label each diagram, consciously reminding yourself of their differences as you do so.

KEY: THE THREE TYPES OF MUSCLE TISSUE					
Type	Striated or Non-striated?	Shape of Fibers— Spindle, Cylindrical, or Spiral and Branching?	Single or Multiple Nucleii?	Under Voluntary or Involuntary Control?	Color
Skeletal					
Cardiac					
Smooth					

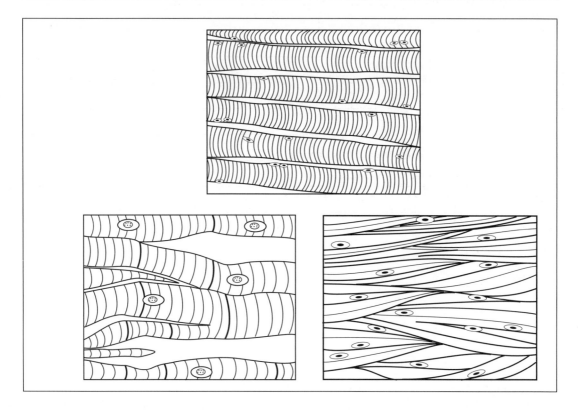

Exercises

1. Word search. Can you find the 13 elements present in the body?

D	M	A	G	N	E	S	I	U	M	O	P
G	A	C	A	L	C	I	U	M	Y	S	O
R	S	H	F	C	F	T	Q	E	T	C	T
A	H	Y	J	I	U	U	E	A	L	H	A
I	L	D	R	H	G	I	H	R	N	E	S
G	Y	R	F	V	O	R	F	B	B	I	S
P	H	O	S	P	H	O	R	U	S	S	I
C	I	G	O	K	P	N	U	N	D	U	U
A	G	E	D	H	F	F	Y	M	W	L	M
R	F	N	I	T	R	O	G	E	N	F	F
B	S	Q	U	F	Q	X	T	T	D	U	C
O	I	R	M	Q	D	Y	W	Q	D	R	F
N	T	R	E	E	I	G	W	F	O	M	K
K	I	O	D	I	N	E	Y	G	O	T	P
C	H	L	O	R	I	N	E	M	U	G	H

2. Fill in the missing words.

   a. _____ compounds do not contain the element carbon. An example of

   such a compound is _____. This compound functions in maintaining the

   _____ of the body by absorbing and giving off large amounts of heat; acting

   as a _____ around organs, bones, ligaments, tendons, and the gastrointestinal

   tract; cushioning and protecting organs such as the _____; and acting as a

   _____ into which many different substances can dissolve and be transported

   around the body.

   b. Organic compounds contain the element _____. Carbohydrates,

   _____, _____, _____ _____ and

   _____ _____ are all examples of important organic compounds

   present in the body.

   c. Carbohydrates contain the elements _____, _____, and oxygen,

   and provide _____ for the body.

    d. Lipids are commonly called _____ and contain the elements _____,

        _____, and _____.

    e. Proteins contain the elements _____, _____, _____, and

        _____, and sometimes _____.

3. **Link each organic compound with its role in the body and write your answers in the spaces given below.**

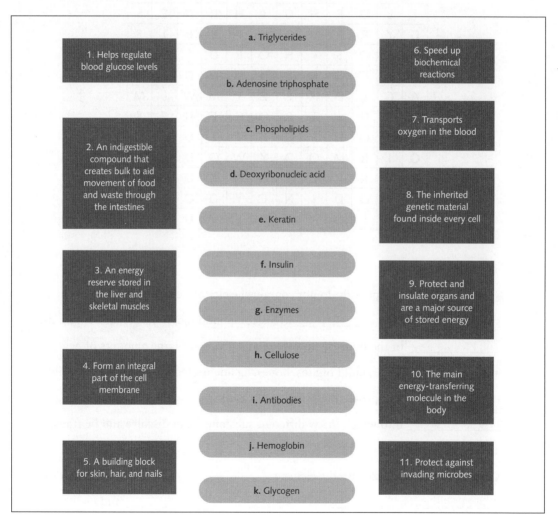

Answers:

1. _____   2. _____   3. _____   4. _____   5. _____   6. _____

7. _____   8. _____   9. _____   10. _____   11. _____

4. **The figure below shows a generalized animal cell. Complete the labeling of this diagram by filling in the blank spaces.**

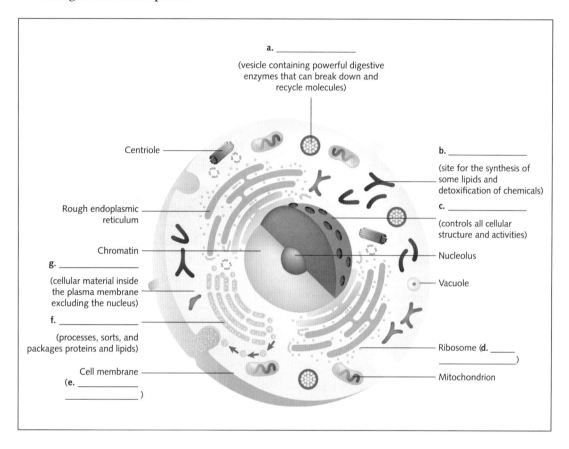

a. _____
(vesicle containing powerful digestive enzymes that can break down and recycle molecules)

Centriole

b. _____
(site for the synthesis of some lipids and detoxification of chemicals)

c. _____
(controls all cellular structure and activities)

Rough endoplasmic reticulum

Nucleolus

Chromatin

g. _____
(cellular material inside the plasma membrane excluding the nucleus)

Vacuole

f. _____
(processes, sorts, and packages proteins and lipids)

Ribosome (d. _____)

Cell membrane
(e. _____)

Mitochondrion

5. **Are the following statements true or false? Write T or F in the spaces provided.**

a. In vesicular transport particles are carried across the plasma membrane in sacs. _____

b. Osmosis is the movement of water from an area of high solute concentration to an area of low solute concentration. _____

c. Simple diffusion is the movement of water only from areas of high concentration to areas of low concentration. _____

d. Somatic cell division takes place when the body needs to replace dead and injured cells or produce new cells for growth. _____

e. Human cells have 23 chromosomes. _____

f. In somatic cell division a single diploid parent cell duplicates itself into two identical daughter cells through a process called meiosis. _____

g. Through the process of mitosis a mother cell divides into two identical daughter cells. _____

h. Cytokinesis occurs during mitosis and is the period in which chromosomes go to the opposite ends of the cell and the mitotic spindle breaks down and disappears. _____

i. Histology is the study of the different types of cells in the body. _____

j. There are four types of tissue in the body: epithelial, connective, muscle, and nervous. _____

6. **Complete the following table on the different tissue types found in the body.**

TYPES OF TISSUE IN THE BODY			
Tissue Type	**Description**	**Function**	**Example**
a.	A loose, soft, and semifluid type of connective tissue containing collagen, elastic, and reticular fibers	Strength, elasticity, and support	Surrounds body organs
Transitional epithelium	**b.**	Stretching and distension	Bladder
Fibrocartilage	Strongest type of cartilage, consisting of cells scattered between bundles of collagen fibers	Support and strength	**c.**
Simple cuboidal epithelium	Single layer of cube-shaped cells	**d.**	Forms ducts of many glands
e.	A single layer of rectangular cells containing cilia	Moving fluid or particles along a passageway	Fallopian tubes
Adipose tissue	An areolar tissue containing many fat cells	**f.**	Subcutaneous layer of the skin
g.	Consists of many freely branching elastic fibers, few cells, and little matrix; has a yellowish color	Stretching and strength	Walls of arteries
Cardiac muscle tissue	A muscle tissue consisting of branched, striated fibers not under conscious control	Pumps blood	**h.**

TYPES OF TISSUE IN THE BODY			
Tissue Type	Description	Function	Example
i.	Wet membranes lining body cavities that open to the exterior	Lubrication, movement, and protection	Respiratory tract
Connective tissue membranes/ synovial membranes	Composed of areolar connective tissue with elastic fibers and fat; secrete synovial fluid	j.	Line cavities of freely movable joints such as the shoulder joint

7. List the general causes of cellular injury.

a. _____

b. _____

c. _____

d. _____

e. _____

f. _____

g. _____

Study groups

Choose five diseases that you need to know in depth. Analyze each of these diseases in terms of what is happening on a cellular level—what is injuring the cell and how is the body responding?

8. If a patient presents with the following generalized signs and symptoms, what disease process should you consider?
   - Nausea
   - Vomiting
   - Diarrhea
   - Fever
   - Weight loss

   Answer: _____

9. List four different treatments available for cancer.

a. _____

b. _____

c. _____

d. _____

Vocabulary test

Complete the table below.

WORD	DEFINITION
Phagocytosis	a. _____
Enzyme	b. _____
Homeostasis	c. _____
Diploid	d. _____
Vesicle	e. _____
Metabolism	f. _____
Somatic cell	g. _____
Gene	h. _____
Solvent	i. _____
Kinetic energy	j. _____
Chromatin	k. _____
Biopsy	l. _____
Ischemia	m. _____
Cytokinesis	n. _____
Cancer	o. _____
Hypoxia	p. _____
Benign	q. _____
Metastasis	r. _____

Multiple-Choice Questions

1. The basic unit of matter is a:
   a. Compound
   b. Chemical
   c. Atom
   d. Element

2. The four major elements of the body are:
   a. Sulfur, molybdenum, oxygen, and nitrogen
   b. Hydrogen, oxygen, nitrogen, and copper
   c. Oxygen, nitrogen, hydrogen, and zinc
   d. Carbon, hydrogen, oxygen, and nitrogen

3. What group of organic compounds includes triglycerides and steroids?
   a. Carbohydrates
   b. Lipids
   c. Proteins
   d. Nucleic acids

4. Which of the following is the main energy-transferring molecule in the body?
   a. ATP
   b. ADP
   c. DNA
   d. RNA

5. Free radicals are:
   a. Molecules that are vital for the proper functioning of the body
   b. Substances that combat or neutralize unstable cells
   c. Molecules that are highly unstable and reactive and that damage cells
   d. Substances that play a role in the growth and development of the body

6. The movement of water across a selectively permeable membrane from an area of high water concentration to an area of low water concentration is called:
   a. Osmosis
   b. Simple diffusion
   c. Active transport
   d. Vesicular transport

7. In a cell, proteins are synthesized in the:
   a. Mitochondria
   b. Lysosomes
   c. Centrosomes
   d. Ribosomes

8. In a cell, ATP is generated in the:
   a. Mitochondria
   b. Lysosomes
   c. Centrosomes
   d. Ribosomes

9. How many chromosomes do you inherit from your father?
   a. 13
   b. 23
   c. 36
   d. 46

10. The time in which a cell grows and prepares itself for division through DNA replication is called:
    a. Mitosis
    b. Meiosis
    c. Interphase
    d. Cytokinesis

11. Which of the following has the stages of mitosis in their correct chronological sequence?
    a. Interphase, prophase, metaphase, anaphase, telophase, interphase
    b. Anaphase, prophase, telophase, interphase, metaphase, anaphase
    c. Telophase, anaphase, prophase, metaphase, interphase, telophase
    d. Metaphase, interphase, prophase, telophase, anaphase, metaphase

12. What type of tissue usually lines hollow organs, cavities, and ducts?
    a. Epithelial
    b. Connective
    c. Muscle
    d. Nervous

13. What type of tissue protects and supports the body and also binds organs together and stores energy reserves?
    a. Epithelial
    b. Connective
    c. Muscle
    d. Nervous

14. The words squamous, cuboidal, columnar, and transitional all describe which type of tissue cells?
    a. Epithelial
    b. Connective
    c. Muscle
    d. Nervous

15. The main function of lymphoid (reticular) tissue is:
    a. Allows for distension
    b. Energy reserve
    c. Support framework
    d. Secretion and absorption

3 The Skin, Hair, and Nails

Review/Self–Study Notes

The skin

The skin is a cutaneous membrane made of two distinct layers, the epidermis and the dermis. When studying the skin it is important to know the difference between these two layers.

1. Complete the table below to highlight the differences between the epidermis and dermis.

Description	Epidermis	Dermis
Where in the skin is this layer found? Is it superficial or deep?		
What type of tissue is this layer composed of?		
What are the main functions of this layer?		
What types of cells does this layer contain?		
How many sub-layers is each layer composed of?		
Write a few words or a short phrase to remind you of this layer.		

Study tip

You may be the type of person who remembers images more easily than words. If you are, then use symbols or images instead of words. For example, when learning the stratum basale/ germinativum in the following exercise, you could draw a seed beginning to germinate. Don't be afraid to have fun—remember, the more personal, colorful, amusing, and fun an image or phrase is the easier you will remember it.

2. The epidermis is composed of five different layers. In the space below draw the different layers of the epidermis, and next to each write a short phrase or draw an image or symbol that will remind you of this layer.

The five layers of the epidermis can also be categorized into two major layers. Write a short description to remind yourself of each of these layers:

- Inner (Malpighian) layer
- Outer layer

3. The dermis is composed of only two layers, the papillary and reticular layers. Write a short phrase to remind you of each layer.

   • Papillary layer _____   • Reticular layer _____

4. Although it is not part of the skin, you need to learn about the subcutaneous layer of tissue beneath the skin. This tissue attaches the reticular layer of the dermis to the underlying organs. What type of tissue is this layer made up of?

   _____

5. There are six main skin types: normal/balanced, oily, dry, mature, combination, and sensitive. In the following chart, draw six different faces and on each face draw in the main characteristics of each skin type. Use lots of colors and your imagination, and have fun!

Normal/balanced	Oily
Dry	Mature
Combination	Sensitive

Study groups

Bring your anatomy and physiology studies to life. Form a group and analyze each other's skin type. Remember to not just look at the skin but also feel it for greasiness, coarseness, or dryness and ask questions about health and lifestyle. Once you have seen and felt the different skin types you won't forget them.

6. Color in and label the following diagram of the skin.

KEY: THE SKIN		
Structure	Function/Description	Color
Epidermis		Only the label is needed here; you will color each layer of the epidermis in a different color
Stratum corneum		
Stratum lucidum		
Stratum granulosum		
Stratum spinosum		
Stratum basale (germinativum)		
Dermis (note: this diagram does not differentiate between the papillary and reticular layers of the dermis, so don't stress about those)		
Subcutaneous layer (hypodermis)		
Hair root (bulb)		
Hair shaft		
Arrector pili muscle		
Sebaceous oil gland		
Sweat gland		
Blood vessels		
Nerves and nerve corpuscles		

Hair (pili)

7. Humans have three different types of hair—lanugo, vellus, and terminal. Complete the table below.

Hair Type	Description	Where Is It Found?
Lanugo		
Vellus		
Terminal		

8. The diagrams below show the basic structure of a hair in longitudinal cross-section. Color and label them.

KEY: THE HAIR		
Structure	Function/Description	Color
Diagram A		
Hair root (bulb)		
Hair shaft		
Sebaceous gland		
Arrector pili muscle		

KEY: THE HAIR		
Diagram B		
Inner medulla		
Middle cortex		
Outer cuticle		

Connective tissue sheath

Inner root sheath

Outer root sheath

A.

B.

9. Using your own words, describe the life cycle of a hair.

_____

_____

_____

_____

_____

_____

Nails

When learning about the nails you might feel overwhelmed by all the different terms you need to learn. Unfortunately, there is no easy way to learn all these terms and you will just have to memorize them. Make up some flash cards to help you remember the following terms:

- Germinal matrix
- Nail bed
- Cuticle
- Eponychium
- Nail plate
- Free edge

- Nail groove
- Nail mantle
- Lunula
- Hyponychium
- Nail wall

10. Now color and label the following diagrams of the nail.

KEY: THE NAIL		
Structure	Function/Description	Color
Diagram A: Finger cross-section		
Germinal matrix		
Nail bed		
Nail plate		
Free edge		
Distal phalanx		
Skin		
Diagram B: Nail		
Nail mantle (fold)		
Cuticle		
Lunula		

KEY: THE NAIL		
Structure	**Function/Description**	**Color**
Diagram B: Nail		
Nail plate		
Nail groove		
Free edge		
Diagram C: Nail anatomy		
Germinal matrix		
Nail bed		
Eponychium		
Hyponychium		

A.

B.

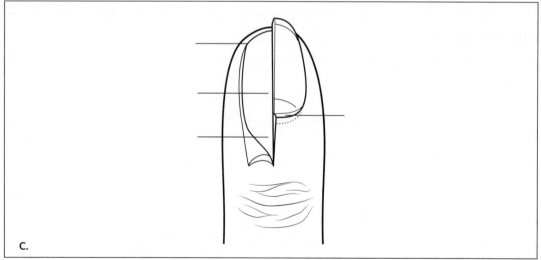

C.

Study groups

Play a game with the flash cards. One person stands up in front of the group and calls out either the term or the definition on the card. The members of the group then compete to call out the correct answer. Whoever calls out the correct answer first wins a point. At the end of the game the person with the most points wins!

Cutaneous glands

Glands are groups of specialized cells that can either secrete beneficial substances or excrete waste products from the body. The main glands associated with the skin are sebaceous and sudoriferous (sweat) glands.

11. **In your own words, write down a simple phrase to remind you of each type of gland.**

    • Sebaceous glands _____

    • Sudoriferous glands _____

12. **Sudoriferous glands can be divided into eccrine and apocrine glands, depending on their location, structure, secretion, and function. Draw spider diagrams or mind maps to help you remember each of them.**

Common pathologies of the skin, hair, and nails

> ### Study tip
> ....
>
> Learn both the clinical and common names of these diseases and disorders and you will notice that you already know many of them. For example, you know what nail biting is—now you just need to learn its clinical name: onychophagy.

13. **As a therapist you will need to have a basic understanding of a wide variety of skin diseases and disorders. Write down a short phrase that will remind you of each of the following. The first one has been completed for you.**

    Abnormal growth disorders:

    • Acrochordon <u>skin tag</u>_____

    • Alopecia _____

    • Keloids _____

    • Psoriasis _____

    • Seborrheic keratoses (senile warts)

      _____

    • Xanthoma _____

    Allergies:

    • Contact dermatitis _____

    • Eczema _____

    • Urticaria (nettle rash or hives) _____

    Bacterial infections of the skin:

    • Carbuncles _____

    • Cellulitis _____

    • Conjunctivitis _____

    • Folliculitis _____

    • Furuncles (boils) _____

    • Hordeolum (stye) _____

    • Impetigo _____

Cancers:

- Basal cell carcinoma (rodent ulcers)

  _____

- Melanoma _____

- Squamous cell carcinoma (prickle-cell cancer) _____

Fungal infections of the skin:

- Candidiasis (thrush or yeast infection)

  _____

- Tinea capitis (scalp ringworm) _____

- Tinea corporis (body ringworm)

  _____

- Tinea pedis (athlete's foot) _____

Infestations of the skin:

- Pediculosis capitis (head lice) _____

- Pediculosis corporis (body lice)

  _____

- Pediculosis pubis (pubic lice) _____

- Scabies (itch mites) _____

Pigmentation disorders:

- Albinism _____

- Chloasma _____

- Dilated capillaries _____

- Ephelides (freckles) _____

- Erythema _____

- Lentigines _____

- Leucoderma _____

- Vascular nevi _____

- Vitiligo _____

- Pressure sores (decubitus ulcers)

  _____

Sebaceous gland disorders:

- Acne rosacea _____

- Acne vulgaris _____

- Comedones (blackheads) _____

- Milia _____

- Seborrhea _____

- Steatomas (sebaceous cysts or wens)

  _____

Sudoriferous (sweat) gland disorders

- Anhidrosis _____

- Bromhidrosis (body odor) _____

- Hyperhidrosis _____

- Miliaria rubra (prickly heat) _____

Viral infections of the skin:

- Herpes simplex (cold sore) _____

- Herpes zoster (shingles) _____

- Rubella (German measles) _____

- Rubeola (measles) _____

- Varicella (chickenpox) _____

- Warts/verrucae _____

Pathologies of the nails:

- Agnail (hang nail) _____

- Anonychia _____

- Beau's lines _____

- Egg-shell nails _____

- Koilonychia (spoon nail) _____
- Leuconychia (white nails or white spots) _____
- Longitudinal furrows _____
- Onychauxis (thick nails) _____
- Onychogryposis (ram's horn nails) _____
- Onychocryptosis (ingrowing nail) _____
- Onycholysis _____
- Onychophagy (nail biting) _____

- Onychoptosis (nail shedding) _____
- Onychorrhexis (brittle nails) _____
- Paronychia (bacterial infection of cuticle) _____
- Pterygium (overgrowth of cuticle) _____
- Severely bruised nail _____
- Tinea unguium (ringworm of the nail) _____

Study tip

Anatomy and physiology is a living subject so when learning it always try to remember you are learning about your own body. You can bring the pathologies of the skin to life by finding people who suffer from these conditions, looking at them, and chatting to them about their condition. It shouldn't be difficult to find people who bite their nails (onychophagy); who have eczema, dermatitis, or psoriasis; or who suffer from cold sores (herpes simplex).

Exercises

1. Red flags: Read the presentations below and circle all those that require referral to a doctor.
   a. Warts growing in clusters on the knees, hands, or fingers
   b. Rash accompanied by fever, nausea, and/or headache
   c. White spots or streaks on the nail
   d. Generalized pruritus of the body
   e. Skin conditions that are infected, blistering, painful, or rapidly worsening
   f. Moles that are changing, itchy, or bleeding
   g. Pruritus of the hand

2. Remember, there are always four things you need to consider when examining a person's skin lesions or moles—ABCD. Write them in the spaces provided.

   A _____

   B _____

   C _____

   D _____

3. List seven functions of the skin.

a. _____

b. _____

c. _____

d. _____

e. _____

f. _____

g. _____

4. The figure below shows the anatomy of the skin. Complete the labeling of this diagram by filling in the blank spaces.

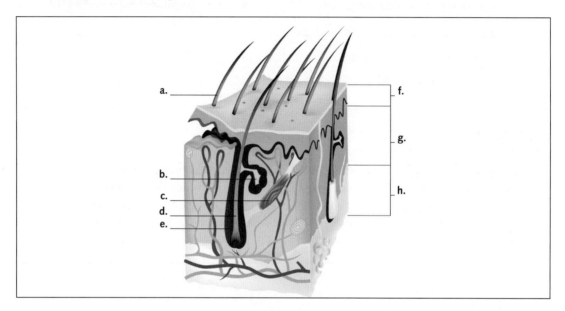

5. Are the following statements true or false? Write T or F in the spaces provided.

a. The skin is composed of two layers—the epidermis, which contains the nerves, blood vessels, sweat glands, and hair roots, and the dermis, which is continuously being worn away. _____

b. The epidermis is composed of keratinized stratified squamous epithelium. _____

c. The dermis is composed of areolar and adipose tissue. _____

d. The dermis is attached to a subcutaneous layer, which anchors the skin to other organs of the body. _____

e. The subcutaneous layer is composed of connective tissue, collagen, and elastic fibers. _____

6. **The skin is made up of a number of different cell types. In the table below, match the cell type to its correct function and write the answers in the spaces provided.**

Cell	Function
1. Adipocytes	**a.** Produce a pigment that contributes to skin color and absorbs ultraviolet light
2. Fibroblasts	**b.** Produce a protein that waterproofs and protects the skin
3. Keratinocytes	**c.** Engulf and destroy bacteria and cell debris through the process of phagocytosis
4. Langerhans cells	**d.** Provide insulation
5. Macrophages	**e.** Function in the sensation of touch
6. Mast cells	**f.** Synthesize collagen, elastic, and reticular fibers
7. Melanocytes	**g.** Function in skin immunity
8. Merkel cells	**h.** Produce histamine during inflammation

Answers:

1. _____ 2. _____ 3. _____ 4. _____ 5. _____ 6. _____ 7. _____ 8. _____

7. **The epidermis is composed of five layers. Put these layers into their correct order, working from the most superficial to the deepest layer.**
   a. Stratum spinosum
   b. Stratum lucidum
   c. Stratum basale
   d. Stratum corneum
   e. Stratum granulosum

   Correct order: _____

8. Complete the following crossword on the anatomy and physiology of the hair and nails.

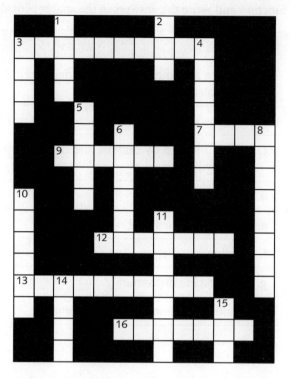

Across

3. A function of both hair and nails (10).
7. Portion of the hair that penetrates into the dermis (4).
9. The soft hair covering a fetus while in the womb (6).
12. The transitional stage in the life cycle of a hair in which a fully grown hair detaches from the matrix (7).
13. An extension of the cuticle from the base of the nail fold (10).
16. The resting stage of the hair growth cycle (7).

Down

1. Another name for the nail mantle (4).
2. Sebaceous _____ glands secrete sebum, which lubricates hair (3).
3. The arrector _____ is the muscle that pulls hairs into a vertical position (4).
4. _____ hairs prevent the inhalation of insects (7).
5. The superficial end of the hair that projects from the surface of the skin (5).
6. The crescent-shaped white area at the proximal end of the nail (6).
8. Type of hair found on the head (8).
10. The growing or active phase of the life cycle of a hair (6).
11. A nipple-shaped projection found in the hair bulb at the base of the follicle (7).
14. The Latin word for "nail" (4).
15. The area lying directly beneath the nail plate (3).

9. **Fill in the missing words.**

   a. The _____ is the supportive layer beneath the epidermis and it can be divided

      into two layers, the _____ layer and the _____ layer.

   b. The _____ layer is an undulating membrane composed of _____

      _____ tissue and _____ fibers. It has nipple-shaped, fingerlike

      projections called _____, which project into the epidermis and contain loops

      of _____, so that diffusion of nutrients and oxygen can take place between

      the dermis and epidermis.

   c. The _____ layer is composed of _____ _____

      _____ tissue and contains both _____ and _____ fibers.

      This layer is the main support structure of the skin and it also contains _____

      follicles, _____, oil _____, ducts of _____ glands, and

      _____ tissue. The _____ layer is attached to the underlying organs

      by the _____ layer, which contains _____ _____ tissue,

      _____ tissue, and nerve endings sensitive to pressure.

10. **Three clients come into your salon and ask you what skin type they have. Next to each description below, give the name of the skin type.**

   a. Susan's skin is flaky with dry patches and a fine texture. When you touch her skin it

      feels papery and you can see that she is aging prematurely, especially around her eyes

      and mouth. Susan's skin type is: _____.

   b. Carl has good skin. It is smooth, even, and blemish-free. When you touch it, it is soft

      and firm and has good elasticity. Carl's skin type is: _____.

   c. Samantha has always had problem skin. Most products make her skin red and

      itchy and she finds it is often dry and chafes easily. She also has dilated capillaries,

      and when you touch her skin it feels unusually warm. Samantha's skin type is:

      _____.

11. **State whether the following are (1) sebaceous, (2) eccrine sudoriferous, or (3) apocrine sudoriferous glands.**

   a. This type of gland excretes waste and helps regulate the body's temperature.

      _____

b. This type of gland is located in the axilla, pubic region, and the areolae of the breasts.
   _____

c. This gland's secretory portion is located in the subcutaneous layer and its duct extends outward through the skin, opening as a pore on the surface of the skin. _____

d. This is an oil gland that usually empties into hair follicles. _____

e. This type of gland secretes a lubricant that prevents excessive evaporation of moisture from the skin. _____

Common pathologies of the skin, hair, and nails

12. Identify the following pathologies.

a. A form of dermatitis that is characterized by itching and redness of the skin. It can be either dry or weeping, can cause scaling and thickening of the skin, and can be caused by either internal or external factors. _____

b. A pus-filled pocket of infection beneath the skin. This bacterial infection is common in people with poor hygiene or a weakened immune system. _____

c. A contagious fungal infection that presents as an itchy, scaly, pink rash on the scalp. It causes patches of hair loss. _____

d. A common fungal infection located between the toes. Its signs and symptoms include scaling, with or without redness and itching. It is easily spread in moist areas where people walk barefoot. _____

e. A pigmentation disorder caused by the overproduction of melanin. It is common in women and can be triggered by hormonal changes such as during pregnancy or when taking the contraceptive pill. It presents as blotchy, brownish patches, usually on the forehead or cheeks or around the lips. _____

f. A pigmentation disorder caused by a lack of melanocytes and characterized by smooth, white patches of skin. _____

g. Common in newborn babies, these are small keratin-filled cysts that commonly appear as white, hard nodules under the skin. They are usually around the eyes or over the cheek and are harmless. _____

h. Caused by a virus, these firm growths are generally painless and can grow in clusters or as isolated growths. They are common on areas that are frequently injured; for example, the knees, face, fingers, and around the nails. When they occur on the feet they can be painful due to the weight of the body on them. _____

i. These are transverse ridges or grooves on the nail plate and usually reflect a temporary retardation of growth due to ill health, a very high temperature, or a zinc deficiency in the body. _____

j. A bacterial infection of the skin surrounding the nails. This is a common infection that can be the result of injury, nail biting, or poor manicure techniques. _____

k. A fungal infection of the nails characterized by thickened and deformed nails. Infected nails may separate from the nail bed, crumble, or flake off.

_____

13. **In the table below, match the clinical name of the disease or disorder to its common name and write the answers in the spaces provided.**

Clinical Name	Common Name
1. Urticaria	**a.** Body ringworm
2. Hordeolum	**b.** Overgrowth of cuticle
3. Candidiasis	**c.** Hives
4. Pediculosis	**d.** Ingrowing nail
5. Tinea corporis	**e.** Measles
6. Ephelides	**f.** Stye
7. Erythema	**g.** Spoon nail
8. Comedones	**h.** Thrush
9. Herpes simplex	**i.** White spots on nail
10. Herpes zoster	**j.** Nail biting
11. Rubeola	**k.** Shingles
12. Varicella	**l.** Redness of skin
13. Koilonychia	**m.** Chickenpox

Clinical Name	Common Name
14. Leuconychia	**n.** Lice
15. Onychocryptosis	**o.** Cold sore
16. Onychophagy	**p.** Freckles
17. Pterygium	**q.** Blackheads

Answers:

1. _____ 2. _____ 3. _____ 4. _____ 5. _____ 6. _____ 7. _____ 8. _____

9. _____ 10. _____ 11. _____ 12. _____ 13. _____ 14. _____ 15. _____

16. _____ 17. _____

Vocabulary test

Complete the table below.

WORD	DEFINITION
a. _____	The transfer of infection from one person to another
b. _____	The process through which the skin is shed
c. _____	The system of the skin and its derivatives
d. _____	The constriction of blood vessels
e. _____	The dilation of blood vessels
Tumor	**f.** _____
Keratinization	**g.** _____
Excoriation	**h.** _____
Cyst	**i.** _____
Phagocytosis	**j.** _____
Fissure	**k.** _____
Wheal (hive)	**l.** _____
Callus	**m.** _____

Multiple-Choice Questions

1. Which of the following statements is correct?
   a. Functions of the skin include excretion, secretion, and movement
   b. Functions of the skin include blood cell production, vitamin D synthesis, and protection
   c. Functions of the skin include sensation, absorption, and heat regulation
   d. Functions of the skin include protection, olfaction, and sensation

2. Although the skin is waterproof, it can still absorb certain substances. These substances include:
   a. Vitamins B and C
   b. Salts
   c. Water
   d. Fat-soluble vitamins

3. Which of the following statements is true?
   a. The skin is a serous membrane
   b. The skin is a cutaneous membrane
   c. The skin is a synovial membrane
   d. The skin is a mucous membrane

4. What is the name of the thin, protective outer layer of the skin?
   a. Dermis
   b. Epidermis
   c. Hypodermis
   d. Subcutaneous layer

5. What is the name of the deepest layer of the epidermis?
   a. Stratum basale
   b. Stratum spinosum
   c. Stratum granulosum
   d. Stratum corneum

6. In which layer of the epidermis are all the cells dead and completely filled with keratin?
   a. Stratum basale
   b. Stratum spinosum
   c. Stratum granulosum
   d. Stratum corneum

7. Through what process are skin cells constantly shed?
   a. Phagocytosis
   b. Keratinization
   c. Desquamation
   d. Vasoconstriction

8. What is the function of the reticular layer of the dermis?
   a. It greatly increases the surface area of the dermis
   b. It contains loops of capillaries so that diffusion of nutrients and oxygen can take place
   c. It acts as the main support structure of the skin
   d. It is the tissue that attaches the skin to the underlying organs

9. A skin that has an oily t-zone yet dry cheeks and neck can be described as:
   a. Balanced
   b. Oily
   c. Dry
   d. Combination

10. Which of the following statements is correct?
    a. Hairs are columns of living cells
    b. Hairs are columns of reproducing cells
    c. Hairs are columns of keratinized dead cells
    d. Hairs are columns of dead cells covered in melanin

11. The area of a nail in which cell division and growth occur is called the:
    a. Germinal matrix
    b. Hyponychium
    c. Nail plate
    d. Lunula

12. The main glands associated with the skin are:
    a. Endocrine and sebaceous glands
    b. Endocrine glands only
    c. Sebaceous and sudoriferous glands
    d. Sudoriferous glands only

13. What type of gland secretes an oily substance called sebum?
    a. Sebaceous
    b. Cutaneous
    c. Endocrine
    d. Sudoriferous

14. What type of infection is tinea corporis?
    a. Bacterial
    b. Fungal
    c. Viral
    d. Yeast

15. What is the term used to describe inflammation or redness of the skin?
    a. Chloasma
    b. Ephelides
    c. Erythema
    d. Lentigines

4 The Skeletal System

Review/Self–Study Notes

Bones

Bones play a vital role in both the structure
and function of the body, and they do far
more than simply forming a skeleton to
support it.

1. **List the functions of the skeletal system,
   and next to each function write a
   sentence showing you understand that
   function.**

   a. _____

   _____

   _____

   _____

   b. _____

   _____

   _____

   _____

   c. _____

   _____

   _____

   _____

   d. _____

   _____

   _____

   _____

   e. _____

   _____

   _____

   _____

   f. _____

   _____

   _____

   _____

   g. _____

   _____

   _____

   _____

2. **To help you remember the different cells
   that make up bone tissue, create a short
   rhyme that demonstrates the following:**
   - Osteoprogenitor cells are the initial
     stem cells, and can develop into
     osteoblasts.
   - Osteoblasts are the cells that form
     bones. They develop into osteocytes.
   - Osteocytes are the mature bone cells
     that maintain the daily activities of
     bone tissue. They are the main cells
     found in bone tissue.
   - Osteoclasts are cells found on the
     surface of bones that resorb or
     destroy bone tissue.

   Rhyme: _____

   _____

   _____

   _____

3. In the table below, list the differences between compact (dense) bone tissue and spongy (cancellous) bone tissue.

Characteristic	Compact (Dense) Bone Tissue	Spongy (Cancellous) Bone Tissue
Basic description		
Basic structure		
Functions		
Location		

4. To help you master your knowledge of the types of bone tissue, color in and label the following diagrams.

KEY: COMPACT BONE TISSUE		
What is the main function of compact bone tissue?		
Where is compact bone tissue found?		
Structure	**Function/Description**	**Color**
Diagram A		
Haversian canal		
Lacunae		
Osteocyte		
Canaliculi		
Lamellae		

KEY: COMPACT BONE TISSUE		
Diagram B		
Osteon (Haversian system)		
Haversian canal		
Lamellae		
Lacunae		
Periosteum		
Volkmann's canals		

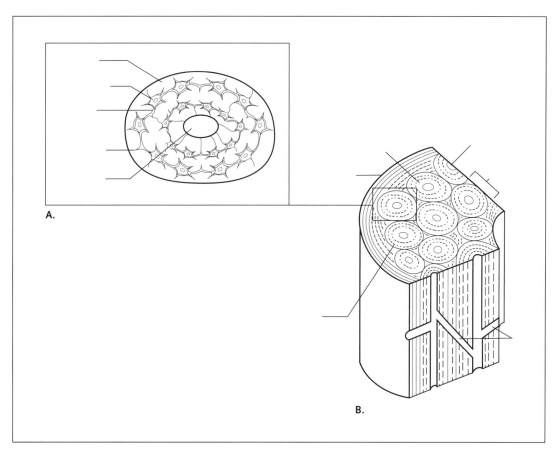

A.

B.

KEY: SPONGY BONE TISSUE		
What is the main function of spongy bone tissue?		
Where is spongy bone tissue found?		
Structure	**Function/Description**	**Color**
Trabeculae		
Lacunae		
Osteocytes		
Red bone marrow		

5. The bones of the body can be classified into the following types—long, short, flat, irregular, and sesamoid. You will find these in the boxes following. Next to each one write its main features and functions. Then work your way through the skeleton, putting all the bones of the skeleton into their correct box. The first one, long bones, has been done for you.

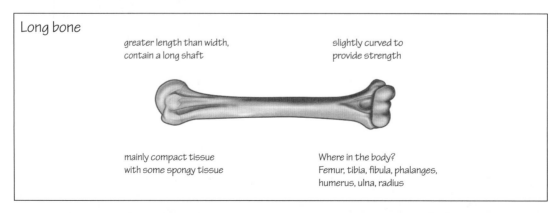

Long bone

greater length than width, contain a long shaft

slightly curved to provide strength

mainly compact tissue with some spongy tissue

Where in the body? Femur, tibia, fibula, phalanges, humerus, ulna, radius

Short bones

Irregular bones

Flat bones

Sesamoid bones

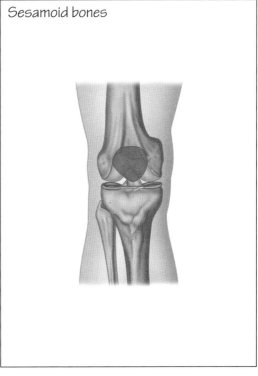

6. Below is a diagram of a long bone. Color and label it.

KEY: STRUCTURE OF A LONG BONE		
Structure	Function/Description	Color
Proximal epiphysis		
Diaphysis		
Distal epiphysis		
Periosteum		
Articular cartilage		
Epiphyseal line		
Spongy bone tissue		
Compact bone tissue		
Medullary cavity (yellow marrow)		

The skeleton

7. Now that you understand the structure, function, and classification of bones, it is time to learn the skeleton. Color in and label the diagrams following, and as you work on each bone repeat its name to yourself a couple of times so that you can memorize it.

Study tip

Before you start, take some time to plan what colors you will need. Try to use the same color for a specific bone on all of the following images. For example, if on the anterior view of the skeleton you choose the color blue for the humerus, then use blue for the humerus in all the other images in which it is depicted.

Also, take note that some structures listed below are part of another structure and therefore should be a similar color—perhaps a shade darker or lighter? These structures are:

- Coracoid process—scapula
- Anterior iliac spine—ilium
- Greater and lesser trochanters—femur
- Medial malleolus—tibia
- Lateral malleolus—fibula
- Mastoid process—temporal bone

KEY: ANTERIOR VIEW OF THE SKELETON			
Structure	Color	Structure	Color
Axial skeleton		*Appendicular skeleton*	
Frontal bone		Radius	
Zygomatic bone		Carpals	
Mandible		Metacarpals	
Maxilla		Phalanges	
Nasal bone		Ilium	
Vertebral column	Not labeled.	Anterior superior iliac spine	
Manubrium		Ischial tuberosity	
Sternum		Pubic symphysis	
Xiphoid process		Femur	
Costal cartilage		Greater trochanter	
First rib		Lesser trochanter	
Ribs 2–10		Patella	
Sacrum		Tibia	
Coccyx		Fibula	
Appendicular skeleton		Medial malleolus	
Clavicle		Lateral malleolus	
Scapula		Tarsals	
Coracoid process		Metatarsals	
Humerus		Phalanges	
Ulna			

KEY: POSTERIOR VIEW OF THE SKELETON				
Structure	Color	Structure	Color
Axial skeleton		*Appendicular skeleton*	
Parietal bone		Humerus	
Occipital bone		Ulna	
Temporal bone		Radius	
Mastoid process		Carpals	
Cervical vertebra: C1, atlas		Metacarpals	
Cervical vertebra: C2, axis		Phalanges	
Cervical vertebrae: C3–C7		Ilium	
Thoracic vertebrae: T1–T12		Posterior iliac spine	
Lumbar vertebrae: L1–L5		Ischial spine	
Sacrum		Ischial tuberosity	
Coccyx		Femur	
Ribs 1–10 (note these are not labeled in the diagram)		Tibia	
Ribs 11–12 (note how these are "floating ribs" and do not attach to the sternum)		Fibula	
Appendicular skeleton		Medial malleolus	
Scapula		Lateral malleolus	
Acromion		Calcaneus	

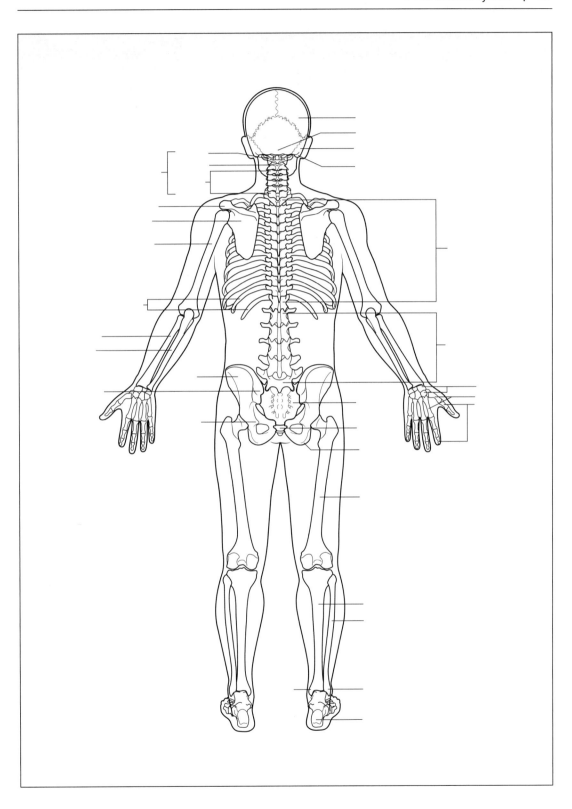

KEY: ANTERIOR VIEW OF THE BONES OF THE SKULL			
Structure	Color	Structure	Color
Frontal bone		Lacrimal bone	
Parietal bone		Ethmoid bone	
Temporal bone		Maxilla	
Sphenoid bone		Mandible	
Zygomatic bone		Vomer	
Nasal bone		Inferior nasal concha (turbinate)	

Note: The palatine bones are not shown in these images.

KEY: LATERAL VIEW OF THE BONES OF THE SKULL			
Structure	Color	Structure	Color
Frontal bone		Zygomatic bone	
Parietal bone		Nasal bone	
Occipital bone		Lacrimal bone	
Temporal bone		Ethmoid bone	
Mastoid process		Maxilla	
Sphenoid bone		Mandible	

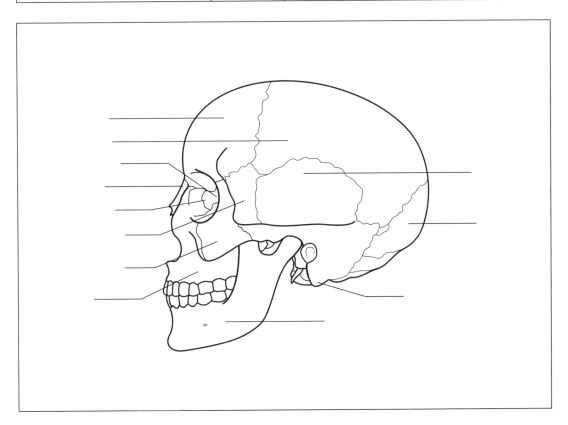

Now, take a highlighter or a red pen and circle the following joints, and in brackets next to the joint write down what *type* of joint it is (for example, the sutures are fibrous joints):

- Sutures of the skull
- Temporomandibular joint

KEY: BONES OF THE UPPER LIMB AND SHOULDER GIRDLE			
Structure	Color	Structure	Color
Diagram A: The upper limb		*Diagram B: The hand*	
Scapula		Trapezoid	
Clavicle		Capitate	
Acromion		Hamate	
Humerus		Pisiform	
Lateral epicondyle		Triquetrum	
Medial epicondyle		Lunate	
Radius		Metacarpals	
Ulna		Proximal phalanges	
Diagram B: The hand		Middle phalanges	
Scaphoid		Distal phalanges	
Trapezium			

Study tip

Remember: Hands Take Crazy Things To Silly Lunch Parties.

Hamate, Trapezium, Capitate, Trapezoid, Triquetrum, Scaphoid, Lunate, Pisiform

Now, take a highlighter or a red pen and circle the following joints, and in brackets next to the joint write down what *type* of joint it is (for example, the elbow joint is a synovial hinge joint):

- Acromioclavicular joint
- Shoulder (glenohumeral) joint
- Elbow joint (composed of the humeroradial joint, humeroulnar joint, and the proximal radioulnar joint)
- Wrist joint
- Midcarpal joint
- Carpometacarpal joints
- Metacarpophalangeal joints
- Interphalangeal joints of the fingers

KEY: LATERAL VIEW OF THE PELVIC GIRDLE, LOWER LIMB, AND FOOT			
Structure	Color	Structure	Color
Ilium		Tibia	
Iliac crest		Fibula	
Anterior superior iliac spine		Talus	
Anterior inferior iliac spine		Calcaneus	
Posterior superior iliac spine		Cuboid	
Ischium		Navicular	
Pubis		Cuneiform (there are three cuneiforms, but in this view only the lateral and intermediate can be seen)	
Femur		Metatarsals	
Patella		Phalanges	

Now, take a highlighter or a red pen and circle the following joints, and in brackets next to the joint write down what *type* of joint it is (for example, the hip joint is a ball-and-socket synovial joint).

- Hip (acetabulofemoral or coxal) joint
- Knee joint (composed of the tibiofemoral and patellofemoral joints)
- Superior tibiofibular joint
- Inferior tibiofibular joint
- Ankle joint (talocrural joint)
- Intertarsal joints
- Tarsometatarsal joints
- Intermetatarsal joints
- Metatarsophalangeal joints
- Interphalangeal joints

Coccyx

KEY: POSTERIOR VIEW OF THE VERTEBRAL COLUMN		
Structure	Number of Vertebrae	Color
Cervical vertebrae	7	
Thoracic vertebrae	12	
Lumbar vertebrae	5	
Sacrum	5 fused vertebrae	
Coccyx	3–4 fused vertebrae	

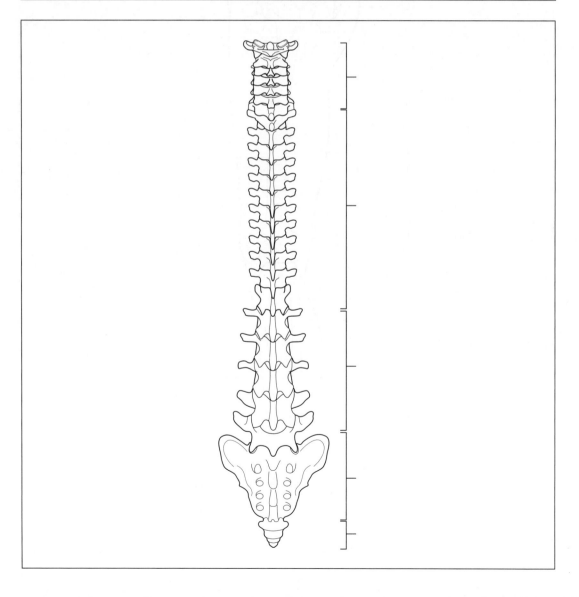

Below are diagrams of the three non-fused types of vertebrae (cervical, thoracic, and lumbar). Color each image in and, as you do so, think about the differences in the shapes and structures of these vertebrae, as noted in the following table. Note, the labels have been left in so that you can really focus on the differences between the vertebrae. Think about *why* the vertebrae differ so much.

DIFFERENCES BETWEEN THE CERVICAL, THORACIC, AND LUMBAR VERTEBRAE			
Feature	Cervical	Thoracic	Lumbar
Size of body	Smallest	Medium	Largest—to bear weight of upper body
Shape of spinous process	Slender	Long and thick	Short and blunt
Are there articular facets for ribs?	No	Yes	No

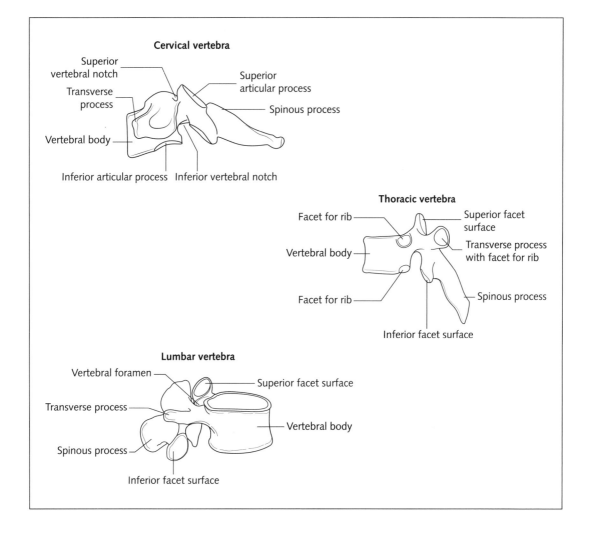

> ### Study tip
> ....
>
> Learn the names of the bones well, because many muscles, blood vessels, and nerves are named
> after the bones along which they run. Study hard now and it will make things easier for you
> later on!

Joints

Joints, or articulations, are the points of contact between bones, and they function in not only
holding bones together but also providing movement.

8. Joints can be classified according to the degree of movement they permit. Complete the
    table below.

Classification	Movement Permitted	Example
Synarthroses		
Amphiarthroses		
Diarthroses		

9. Joints can also be classified according to their structure. Complete the table below.

Classification	Structure	Example
Fibrous		
Cartilaginous		
Synovial		

10. Synovial joints predominate in the limbs of the body and allow for a great variety of movement. Although there are different types of synovial joints, they share common features. To remind yourself of these features, color and label the diagram below.

KEY: SYNOVIAL JOINT		
Structure	**Function/Description**	**Color**
Bone		
Periosteum		
Hyaline cartilage		
Ligament		
Joint capsule		
Synovial membrane		
Synovial fluid		

11. Synovial joints permit a wide range of movements, all of which are listed below. Next to each movement write a few words or a short phrase to remind you of it.

- Flexion _____
- Extension _____
- Hyperextension _____
- Abduction _____
- Adduction _____
- Circumduction _____
- Rotation _____
- Medial (internal) rotation _____
- Lateral (external) rotation _____
- Pronation _____
- Supination _____
- Inversion _____
- Eversion _____
- Dorsiflexion _____
- Plantar flexion _____

12. There are a number of different types of synovial joints, whose names tend to describe them. In the spaces provided, draw a symbol or image that will remind you of each type of synovial joint. Next to the symbol, list or draw the movements it permits and give an example of the joint.

Gliding (plane)	Hinge
Pivot	Condyloid
Saddle	Ball-and-socket (spheroidal)

Make your own poster

This will be a big project for you and will take a lot of time—but will definitely be worth the effort.

Take a large piece of plain white cardboard (preferably A1). Hand draw in the entire skeleton. Spend time on each and every bone, thinking about its shape, size, and relation to the rest of the body. Don't worry if you aren't an artist. It is just important that you do it yourself and really think about it as you do it.

Make it as large as possible and on a piece of cardboard, because you will add to it as you revise each system of the body—so you want it to be large, clear, and strong.

Now:

- Color in and label each bone, and in brackets next to the name write what type of bone it is (long, short, flat, irregular, or sesamoid).
- Label each joint, and in brackets next to the name write what type of joint it is (fibrous, cartilaginous, or synovial). If it is a synovial joint then write down its classification (gliding, hinge, pivot, condyloid, saddle, ball-and-socket).
- Focusing on the femur, label the structures of a long bone (epiphysis, metaphysis, and diaphysis).

Take this poster and stick it on a wall in your house. Every time you look at the poster learn just one bone or one joint. Look at the poster as often as you can! Remember, if you learn the names of the bones and joints really well, it will help you learn the rest of your anatomy.

Common pathologies of the skeletal system

13. **In the spaces provided write a few words or a short phrase that will remind you of the disease or disorder listed. The first one has been done for you.**

   Pathologies of the skeletal system:

   - Osteoarthritis <u>wear and tear,</u>
     <u>degeneration of cartilage, spurs in joint</u>
   - Psoriatic arthritis _____
   - Rheumatoid arthritis _____
   - Bunion _____
   - Bursitis _____
   - Dislocation (luxation) _____
   - Gout _____
   - Osteogenesis imperfecta (brittle bone disease) _____
   - Osteomalacia/rickets _____
   - Osteoporosis _____
   - Paget's disease _____
   - Sprain _____
   - Torn cartilage _____

Fractures:

   - Simple or closed fracture _____
   - Compound or open fracture _____
   - Comminuted fracture _____
   - Impacted fracture _____
   - Complicated fracture _____
   - Greenstick fracture _____
   - Stress fracture _____

Pathologies of the spine:

   - Cervical spondylosis _____
   - Kyphosis _____
   - Lordosis _____
   - Prolapsed intervertebral disc (PID)
     _____
   - Scoliosis _____
   - Spinal stenosis _____
   - Spondylitis _____
   - Temporomandibular joint disorder
     _____
   - Whiplash injury _____

Disorders of the feet:

   - Club foot (talipes equinovarus) _____
   - Hammer toes _____
   - Heel spur _____
   - Pes cavus (high arches) _____
   - Pes planus (flat foot) _____

Exercises

1. **Word search. Can you find six functions of the skeletal system?**

D	K	E	I	L	N	J	H	B	I	F	M	M	G	I
A	S	A	M	G	E	K	X	J	D	W	F	O	U	G
W	E	I	I	U	J	F	D	X	B	C	M	D	L	L
A	B	E	N	E	R	G	Y	S	T	O	R	A	G	E
S	E	U	E	I	O	S	X	D	Q	Z	E	D	Z	E
I	H	D	R	O	O	U	A	S	G	E	O	L	G	S
K	D	F	A	P	K	P	C	P	E	E	L	K	Y	Z
G	F	P	L	J	N	P	Y	R	D	J	T	H	M	U
V	H	A	H	E	M	O	P	O	I	E	S	I	S	T
N	C	U	O	G	A	R	U	T	G	L	I	Y	S	J
O	C	G	M	E	S	T	J	E	E	F	Y	U	A	I
U	O	D	E	S	Q	S	M	C	J	S	O	I	T	T
L	U	O	O	G	E	A	O	T	Z	J	G	G	F	O
N	D	J	S	V	F	G	E	I	L	G	D	X	S	I
C	K	T	T	M	A	O	M	O	V	E	M	E	N	T
S	L	E	A	B	I	T	A	N	D	S	A	W	O	A
R	F	E	S	D	F	J	X	G	X	Z	E	L	T	D
E	H	H	I	S	E	N	I	T	S	A	D	I	Q	S
S	A	N	S	Q	G	E	Y	O	B	Q	C	Y	A	E

2. **Fill in the missing words.**

   a. _____ is the study of bone. Bone tissue is also called _____ tissue, and it is a _____ tissue.

   b. Bone tissue is composed of water, protein, fibers, and _____ salts. The fibers of bone tissue are made of _____, which gives bones their tensile strength. The salts of bone tissue are mainly _____ carbonate and a crystallized compound called _____. These salts give bone its _____.

3. There are two different types of bone tissue. What are they?

   a. _____

   b. _____

4. Bones can generally be classified into five different types. The figure below gives examples of each of these. In the spaces provided, label each type of bone.

5. **The table below details the structure of a long bone. Match the term to its correct description and write the answers in the space provided.**

Term	Description
1. Diaphysis	**a.** Membrane covering the space inside the diaphysis
2. Epiphysis	**b.** Area where bone shaft joins bone end
3. Metaphysis	**c.** Membrane covering the bone
4. Epiphyseal plate	**d.** Central shaft of bone
5. Periosteum	**e.** Space inside diaphysis
6. Endosteum	**f.** End of bone
7. Medullary (marrow) cavity	**g.** Layer of cartilage that allows bone to grow in length

Answers:

1. _____ 2. _____ 3. _____ 4. _____ 5. _____ 6. _____ 7. _____

6. **Fill in the gaps.**

   The _____ skeleton supports and protects the major organs of the body, while the _____ skeleton forms the upper and lower extremities and their girdles.

7. **Give the correct number of vertebrae for each section of the spine.**

   a. Cervical vertebrae _____

   b. Thoracic vertebrae _____

   c. Lumbar vertebrae _____

   d. Sacral vertebrae _____

   e. Coccygeal vertebrae _____

8. **Give the names of the following bones:**

   a. This bone supports the tongue and provides attachment for some of the muscles of the neck and pharynx. _____

   b. This is the breastbone. _____

   c. There are 12 pairs of these bones and they are located in the thorax. _____

9. **Listed below are the bones of the hands and feet. Connect the name of the bone to the area to which it belongs.**

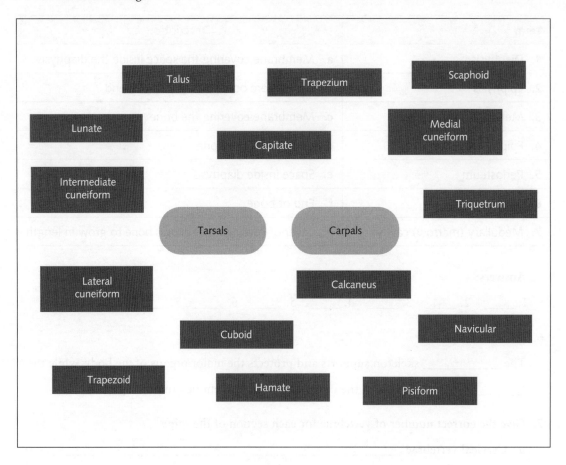

10. **Are the following statements true or false? Write T or F in the spaces provided.**

   a. The bones of the feet can be arranged into four arches. These are the medial longitudinal arch, intermediate longitudinal arch, lateral longitudinal arch, and the transverse arch. _____

   b. A ligament is a band of connective tissue that attaches bones to bones. _____

   c. Diarthrotic joints are immovable joints. _____

   d. The coronal suture is an example of a synarthrotic joint. _____

   e. In a synovial joint, the synovial cavity is the space that separates the articulating bones. _____

   f. Synovial fluid is found between fibrous joints. _____

11. **In the gaps provided, give the correct term for each of the following movements.**

    a. If you bring your chin down to your throat, you are _____ your neck.

    b. When doing star jumps, if you swing your arms up and away from your body you are _____ them.

    c. When turning your palms anteriorly, you are _____ them.

    d. You _____ your arms when swinging them in a large circular movement as if you are warming up your shoulders.

12. **Below are examples of different types of synovial joints. Give the name of each joint type.**

    a. Wrist joint _____

    b. Elbow joint _____

    c. Thumb joint _____

    d. Joint between the axis and atlas _____

    e. Sacroiliac joint _____

    f. Shoulder joint _____

13. **Organize the following bones into their correct sequence, starting proximal and ending distal.**

    a. Metacarpal bones, proximal phalanges, humerus, carpal bones, distal phalanges, radius and ulna, middle phalanges.

    Sequence: _____

    _____

    b. Proximal phalanges, patella, metatarsal bones, tarsal bones, middle phalanges, fibula and tibia, distal phalanges, femur.

    Sequence: _____

    _____

Common pathologies of the skeletal system

14. **Which of the following are NOT considered red flags?**
    a. Joint pain accompanied by stiffness
    b. Joint pain accompanied by fever
    c. Joint pain accompanied by cellulitis
    d. Joint pain accompanied by swelling

15. **Identify the following pathologies of the skeletal system.**

   a. The clinical term for a herniated or slipped disc is a _____ _____ _____, or PID.

   b. _____ _____ is an autoimmune disease in which the body attacks its own cartilage and joint lining. It is characterized by inflammation, swelling, pain, and loss of function of joints and is thought to be hereditary.

   c. A _____ fracture is a fracture that only occurs in children and involves an incomplete break or crack in the bone. The bone then bends.

   d. The disease _____ usually affects men in middle age or older and it involves the build-up of uric acid and its salts in the blood and joints.

   e. An exaggerated thoracic curve of the spine is called _____.

   f. The disease _____ is common in elderly and post-menopausal women and is a progressive disease in which bones lose their density and become brittle and prone to fractures.

   g. An exaggerated lumbar curvature of the spine is called _____.

   h. Painful, rigid toes that are fixed in a contracted position and cannot be straightened are called _____ _____.

   i. The clinical term for high arches is _____ _____.

   j. A lateral curvature of the spine is called _____.

Vocabulary test

Complete the table below.

WORD	DEFINITION
Tendon	a. _____
Ossification	b. _____
Ligament	c. _____
Hemopoiesis	d. _____
Articulation	e. _____
Sinus	f. _____

WORD	DEFINITION
Axial skeleton	g. _____
Diaphysis	h. _____
Demineralization	i. _____
Osteoclasts	j. _____
Menisci	k. _____
Synarthrosis	l. _____

Multiple-Choice Questions

1. **Which of the following are all functions of the skeletal system?**
   a. Movement, shape, and vitamin D synthesis
   b. Hemopoiesis, protection, and support
   c. Mineral homeostasis, heat generation, and gaseous exchange
   d. Blood cell production, energy storage, and waste elimination

2. **The production of blood cells and platelets takes place in:**
   a. Red bone marrow
   b. Yellow bone marrow
   c. The heart
   d. The liver

3. **Mature cells that maintain the daily activities of bone tissue are called:**
   a. Osteoprogenitor cells
   b. Osteoblasts
   c. Osteoclasts
   d. Osteocytes

4. **A hard bone tissue that is composed of a basic structural unit called an osteon, or Haversian system, is:**
   a. Compact bone tissue
   b. Spongy bone tissue
   c. Immature bone tissue
   d. Mature bone tissue

5. **What is the name of the process through which most bones are formed?**
   a. Remodeling
   b. Desquamation
   c. Ossification
   d. Demineralization

6. **Which of the following statements is not true?**
   a. Bone is a dynamic, living tissue that is constantly changing, repairing, and reshaping itself
   b. New bone tissue constantly replaces old, worn-out, or injured bone tissue
   c. Bones are dead materials that support and protect the body and allow for movement
   d. Aging causes bone to lose calcium and other minerals from its matrix

7. Which of the following are all different types of bones?
   a. Long, flat, short, and sesamoid
   b. Long, short, broad, and bursae
   c. Bursae, irregular, flat, and broad
   d. Broad, short, sesamoid, and long

8. An example of a long bone is the:
   a. Patella
   b. Scapula
   c. Triquetrum
   d. Femur

9. What type of bone is a vertebra?
   a. Flat
   b. Short
   c. Irregular
   d. Broad

10. Which of the following statements is true?
    a. Flat bones act as areas of attachment for skeletal muscles and also provide protection
    b. Long bones are hard and straight and function in protection
    c. Bursae are complex bones that act as areas of attachment for skeletal muscles
    d. Sesamoid bones are long and slightly curved to provide strength for locomotion

11. In an adult bone, where is yellow bone marrow found?
    a. Epiphysis
    b. Diaphysis
    c. Periosteum
    d. Medullary cavity

12. Which of the following bones are all categorized as part of the axial skeleton?
    a. Hyoid, ribs, and femur
    b. Sternum, vertebrae, and maxilla
    c. Auditory ossicles, ulna, and pisiform
    d. Tibia, mandible, and phalanges

13. What is the name of the two tiny bones that form the medial wall of the eye orbit?
    a. Maxillae
    b. Lacrimals
    c. Temporals
    d. Parietals

14. What is the correct name for the lower jaw bone?
    a. Sphenoid
    b. Ethmoid
    c. Maxilla
    d. Mandible

15. Which of the following are all bones of the hand?
    a. Trapezoid, lunate, navicular, pisiform
    b. Cuboid, trapezium, capitate, hamate
    c. Calcaneus, cuneiform, pisiform, hamate
    d. Capitate, hamate, scaphoid, lunate

5 The Muscular System

Review/Self–Study Notes

The essential function of all muscles is to shorten themselves, or contract. In doing so, they are able to perform a variety of functions in the body.

1. List the functions of the muscular system.

   * _____

   * _____

   * _____

   * _____

   * _____

   * _____

2. There are three types of muscle tissue in the body—skeletal, cardiac, and smooth (visceral). Each type of muscle has a specific anatomy, location, and function. Make up a mnemonic or draw an image for each muscle type so that you will always be able to remember the following information:
   * **Skeletal muscle:** Striated fibers; attached to bones, skin, or other muscles; functions in locomotion, movements of lymph and venous blood, posture, and heat production; under voluntary control

     Mnemonic: _____

   * **Cardiac muscle:** Striated fibers; forms most of the heart, pumps blood, and helps regulate blood pressure; under involuntary control

     Mnemonic: _____

   * **Smooth (visceral) muscle:** Non-striated fibers; forms walls of hollow internal structures; moves substances through tracts and regulates organ volume; under involuntary control

     Mnemonic: _____

3. The figure below shows the different connective tissues associated with a skeletal muscle. Color and label it.

KEY: SKELETAL MUSCLE TISSUE		
Structure	Function/Description	Color
Bone		
Tendon		
Muscle		
Epimysium (fascia)		
Perimysium		
Fascicle		
Fasciculi (encased by perimysium)		
Endomysium (between muscle fibers)		
Muscle fiber		
Nuclei		
Capillaries		
Sarcolemma (cell membrane)		
Sarcoplasmic reticulum		
Transverse tubule		
Mitochondrion		
Myofibrils		

KEY: SKELETAL MUSCLE TISSUE		
Structure	**Function/Description**	**Color**
Sarcomere		
Actin myofilament		
Myosin myofilament		

4. In your own words, describe how a muscle contracts and relaxes. Make sure you include the following terms or details and cross each one off the list as you write about it. See if you can make a drawing to explain it as well.

- Sarcomere
- Thick filament
- Thin filament
- Myosin
- Myosin heads/cross-bridges
- Actin
- Myosin-binding site
- Elastic filaments
- A-band
- I-band
- Z-disc
- Sliding-filament mechanism
- ATP
- Nerve impulse
- Muscle action potential
- Acetylcholine
- Calcium
- Power-stroke

5. Physical activities include two types of contraction—isotonic and isometric. Complete the table below, which highlights the differences between these two types of contraction.

Description	Isotonic	Isometric
Does muscle shorten?		
Is movement created?		
Function of contraction?		
Write a few words or a short phrase to remind you of this type of contraction.		

Study groups

....

Remember that when learning anatomy and physiology you are learning about yourself. So bring the subject to life by performing the different types of muscular contractions. One person in the group can perform the following types of contractions: isotonic (concentric and eccentric) and isometric. As the person performs each action the other members of the group need to say what type of contraction is being performed.

6. **Muscles need energy in the form of ATP to contract, and they gain this through either the phosphagen system or glycolysis. Write a short phrase or a few words to describe each of the following processes:**

   • The phosphagen system _____

   • Glycolysis _____

   • Anaerobic glycolysis _____

   • Aerobic respiration _____

7. **Three types of muscle fibers exist—slow oxidative, fast oxidative, and fast glycolytic. Write a mnemonic to remind you of the characteristics of each.**
   • **Slow oxidative:** Red, small, good oxygen supply, generate ATP aerobically and split it slowly, resistant to fatigue, plentiful in muscles of endurance or posture

   Mnemonic: _____

   • **Fast oxidative:** Red, medium sized, good oxygen supply, generate ATP aerobically and split it quickly, less resistant to fatigue, plentiful in muscles for walking and running

   Mnemonic: _____

   • **Fast glycolytic:** White, large, poor oxygen supply, generate ATP anaerobically and split it very fast, fatigue easily, plentiful in muscles for fast movements

   Mnemonic: _____

8. **Define the following:**

   • Origin _____

   • Insertion _____

   • Prime mover (agonist) _____

- Antagonist _____
- Synergist _____
- Fixator (stabilizer) _____

9. Following are diagrams of the muscles of the body for you to color and label. As you color each muscle, really think about its origin, insertion, nerve, and action. Repeat these to yourself as you color the muscle. To help you complete this task, refer to chapter 5 of *Anatomy, Physiology, and Pathology* (Hull, 2023). Also, remember to think about the colors and choose them wisely so that the same muscle is the same color on all the different diagrams. Finally, some muscles could appear in more than one section, but have been included only once to avoid repetition.

KEY: MUSCLES OF THE HEAD AND NECK		
Muscle	**Details**	**Color**
Occipitofrontalis	Origin: Insertion: Nerve: Action:	
Temporalis	Origin: Insertion: Nerve: Action:	
Orbicularis oculi	Origin: Insertion: Nerve: Action:	
Procerus	Origin: Insertion: Nerve: Action:	
Nasalis	Origin: Insertion: Nerve: Action:	
Zygomaticus major	Origin: Insertion: Nerve: Action:	
Zygomaticus minor	Origin: Insertion: Nerve: Action:	
Masseter	Origin: Insertion: Nerve: Action:	

KEY: MUSCLES OF THE HEAD AND NECK		
Muscle	**Details**	**Color**
Buccinator	Origin: Insertion: Nerve: Action:	
Levator labii superioris	Origin: Insertion: Nerve: Action:	
Orbicularis oris	Origin: Insertion: Nerve: Action:	
Depressor labii inferioris	Origin: Insertion: Nerve: Action:	
Depressor anguli oris	Origin: Insertion: Nerve: Action:	
Platysma	Origin: Insertion: Nerve: Action:	
Mentalis	Origin: Insertion: Nerve: Action:	
Sternocleidomastoid	Origin: Insertion: Nerve: Action:	
Anterior scalene	Origin: Insertion: Nerve: Action:	
Middle scalene	Origin: Insertion: Nerve: Action:	
Posterior scalene	Origin: Insertion: Nerve: Action:	
Longissimus capitis	Origin: Insertion: Nerve: Action:	

KEY: MUSCLES OF THE TRUNK		
Muscle	**Details**	**Color**
Anterior view		
Pectoralis major	Origin: Insertion: Nerve: Action:	
Rectus abdominis	Origin: Insertion: Nerve: Action:	
External oblique	Origin: Insertion: Nerve: Action:	

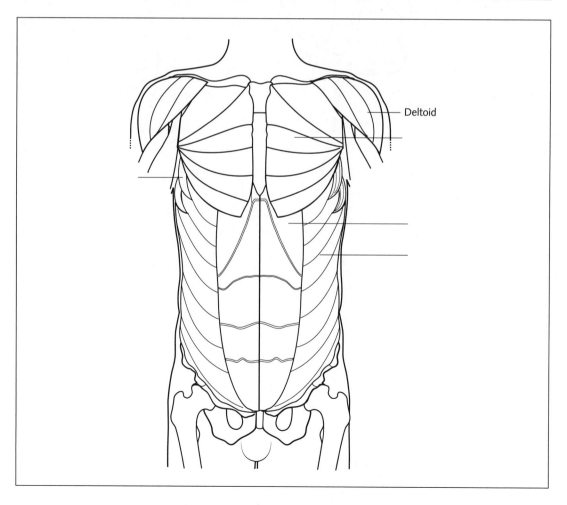

Deltoid

KEY: MUSCLES OF THE TRUNK		
Muscle	**Details**	**Color**
Posterior view		
Superficial extrinsic back muscles		
Latissimus dorsi	Origin: Insertion: Nerve: Action:	

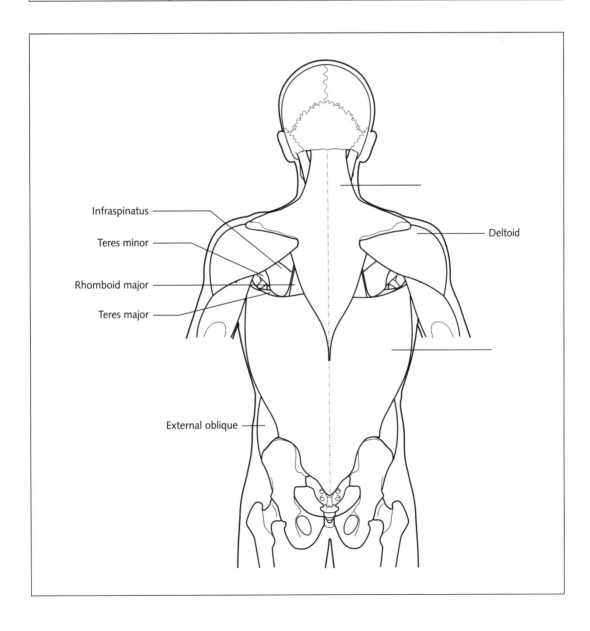

Infraspinatus

Teres minor

Rhomboid major

Teres major

Deltoid

External oblique

KEY: MUSCLES OF THE TRUNK		
Muscle	Details	Color
Posterior view		
Intrinsic back muscles—superficial layer		
Splenius capitis Note: Not shown	Origin: Insertion: Nerve: Action:	
Splenius cervicis Note: Not shown	Origin: Insertion: Nerve: Action:	
Intrinsic back muscles—intermediate layer—erector spinae (sacrospinalis) muscles		
Iliocostalis cervicis	Origin: Insertion: Nerve: Action:	
Iliocostalis thoracis	Origin: Insertion: Nerve: Action:	
Iliocostalis lumborum	Origin: Insertion: Nerve: Action:	
Longissimus capitis	Origin: Insertion: Nerve: Action:	
Longissimus thoracis	Origin: Insertion: Nerve: Action:	
Longissimus lumborum Note: Not shown	Origin: Insertion: Nerve: Action:	
Spinalis capitis	Origin: Insertion: Nerve: Action:	

KEY: MUSCLES OF THE TRUNK		
Muscle	Details	Color
Posterior view		
Spinalis cervicis	Origin: Insertion: Nerve: Action:	
Spinalis thoracis **Note:** Not shown	Origin: Insertion: Nerve: Action:	
Intrinsic back muscles—deep layer—transversospinalis muscles		
Semispinalis capitis	Origin: Insertion: Nerve: Action:	
Semispinalis cervicis	Origin: Insertion: Nerve: Action:	
Semispinalis thoracis	Origin: Insertion: Nerve: Action:	
Interspinales	Origin: Insertion: Nerve: Action:	
Rotatores	Origin: Insertion: Nerve: Action:	
Multifidus	Origin: Insertion: Nerve: Action:	
Intertransversarii	Origin: Insertion: Nerve: Action:	

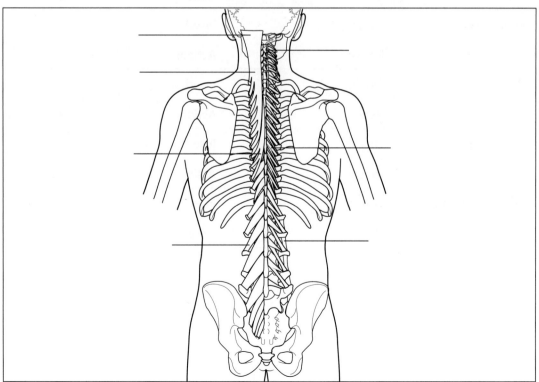

KEY: MUSCLES OF THE SHOULDER		
Muscle	Details	Color
Posterior view		
Upper trapezius	Origin: Insertion: Nerve: Action:	
Middle trapezius	Origin: Insertion: Nerve: Action:	
Levator scapulae	Origin: Insertion: Nerve: Action:	
Supraspinatus	Origin: Insertion: Nerve: Action:	
Infraspinatus	Origin: Insertion: Nerve: Action:	

Spine of scapula

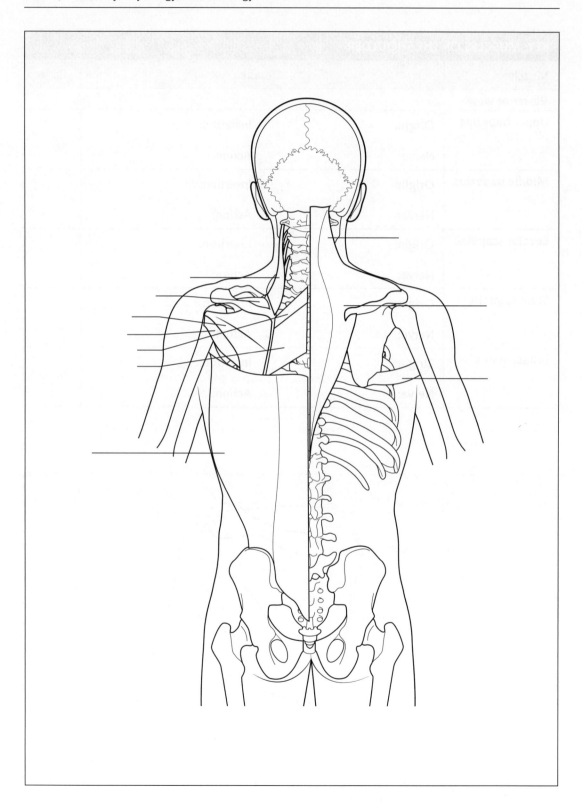

KEY: MUSCLES OF THE SHOULDER		
Muscle	Details	Color
Posterior view		
Teres minor	Origin: Insertion: Nerve: Action:	
Teres major	Origin: Insertion: Nerve: Action:	
Rhomboid minor	Origin: Insertion: Nerve: Action:	
Rhomboid major	Origin: Insertion: Nerve: Action:	
Anterior view		
Deltoid	Origin: Insertion: Nerve: Action:	
Pectoralis major	Origin: Insertion: Nerve: Action:	
Subclavius	Origin: Insertion: Nerve: Action:	
Pectoralis minor	Origin: Insertion: Nerve: Action:	
Coracobrachialis	Origin: Insertion: Nerve: Action:	
Serratus anterior	Origin: Insertion: Nerve: Action:	
Subscapularis	Origin: Insertion: Nerve: Action:	

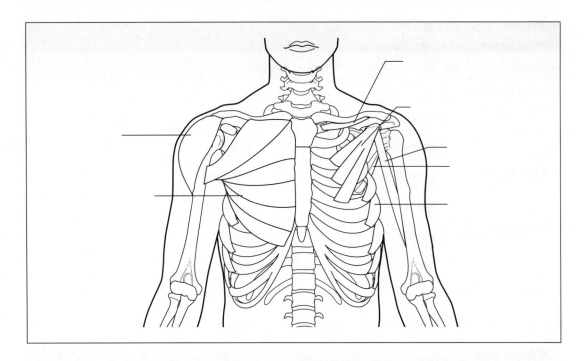

KEY: MUSCLES OF THE ARM AND FOREARM			
Muscle	**Details**		**Color**
Biceps brachii	Origin:	Insertion:	
	Nerve:	Action:	
Brachialis	Origin:	Insertion:	
	Nerve:	Action:	
Brachioradialis	Origin:	Insertion:	
	Nerve:	Action:	
Pronator teres	Origin:	Insertion:	
	Nerve:	Action:	
Triceps brachii	Origin:	Insertion:	
	Nerve:	Action:	

KEY: MUSCLES OF THE ARM AND FOREARM			
Muscle	Details		Color
Anconeus	Origin:	Insertion:	
	Nerve:	Action:	
Flexor carpi radialis	Origin:	Insertion:	
	Nerve:	Action:	
Palmaris longus	Origin:	Insertion:	
	Nerve:	Action:	
Flexor carpi ulnaris	Origin:	Insertion:	
	Nerve:	Action:	
Flexor pollicis longus	Origin:	Insertion:	
	Nerve:	Action:	
Flexor digitorum superficialis	Origin:	Insertion:	
	Nerve:	Action:	
Extensor carpi ulnaris	Origin:	Insertion:	
	Nerve:	Action:	
Extensor digiti minimi	Origin:	Insertion:	
	Nerve:	Action:	
Extensor digitorum	Origin:	Insertion:	
	Nerve:	Action:	
Extensor carpi radialis brevis	Origin:	Insertion:	
	Nerve:	Action:	
Extensor carpi radialis longus	Origin:	Insertion:	
	Nerve:	Action:	

Anterior view

Posterior view

KEY: MUSCLES OF THE HIP AND THIGH

Muscle	Details		Color
Gluteus medius	Origin:	Insertion:	
	Nerve:	Action:	
Gluteus maximus	Origin:	Insertion:	
	Nerve:	Action:	
Tensor fasciae latae	Origin:	Insertion:	
	Nerve:	Action:	
Sartorius	Origin:	Insertion:	
	Nerve:	Action:	
Quadriceps: Vastus lateralis	Origin:	Insertion:	
	Nerve:	Action:	
Quadriceps: Rectus femoris	Origin:	Insertion:	
	Nerve:	Action:	
Quadriceps: Vastus medialis	Origin:	Insertion:	
	Nerve:	Action:	
Pectineus	Origin:	Insertion:	
	Nerve:	Action:	
Adductor brevis	Origin:	Insertion:	
	Nerve:	Action:	
Adductor longus	Origin:	Insertion:	
	Nerve:	Action:	
Adductor magnus	Origin:	Insertion:	
	Nerve:	Action:	

KEY: MUSCLES OF THE HIP AND THIGH		
Muscle	Details	Color
Gracilis	Origin: Insertion: Nerve: Action:	
Hamstrings: Semitendinosus	Origin: Insertion: Nerve: Action:	
Hamstrings: Semimembranosus	Origin: Insertion: Nerve: Action:	
Hamstrings: Biceps femoris	Origin: Insertion: Nerve: Action:	
Fibularis longus	Origin: Insertion: Nerve: Action:	
Fibularis brevis	Origin: Insertion: Nerve: Action:	
Tibialis anterior	Origin: Insertion: Nerve: Action:	
Soleus	Origin: Insertion: Nerve: Action:	
Gastrocnemius	Origin: Insertion: Nerve: Action:	
Extensor digitorum longus **Note:** Not shown	Origin: Insertion: Nerve: Action:	

Anterior view

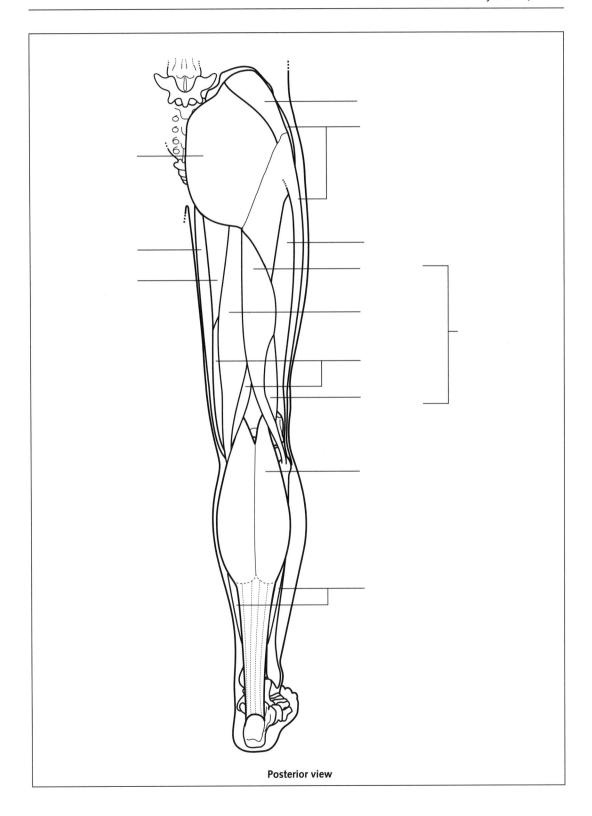

Posterior view

Add to your poster

Take the poster you made when studying the skeletal system and add the muscles to it. The best way to add the muscles is by drawing each individual muscle on very thin paper such as tracing paper or baking paper, cutting the muscle out and sticking it onto the correct bones—be very aware of the size of the muscle and the correct origins and insertions. On top of each muscle you can write its name as well as the major actions it performs.

Study tip

Once again, bring your anatomy and physiology studies to life by working through the muscles on your own body. As you learn a particular muscle, find it on your body. Try to feel it and find where it originates and inserts. Try to contract the muscle so that you can learn its basic actions.

Common pathologies of the muscular system

10. As a therapist you will need to have a basic understanding of a wide variety of muscle diseases and disorders. Write down a short phrase that will remind you of each of the following.

    Diseases and disorders of muscles, bursae, and tendons:

    • Fibromyalgia _____

    • Fibrositis (muscular rheumatism)

    _____

    • Ganglion cyst _____

    • Muscular dystrophies _____

    • Myasthenia gravis _____

    • Poliomyelitis (polio) _____

    • Rupture _____

    • Spasm _____

    • Strain _____

    • Tetanus (lockjaw) _____

    Sports injuries and repetitive strain injury (RSI):

    • Carpal tunnel syndrome _____

    • Frozen shoulder _____

    • Golfer's elbow (medial epicondylitis)

    _____

    • Housemaid's knee (prepatellar

    bursitis) _____

    • Shin splints _____

    • Tendonitis _____

    • Tennis elbow (lateral epicondylitis)

    _____

Exercises

1. Complete the crossword below.

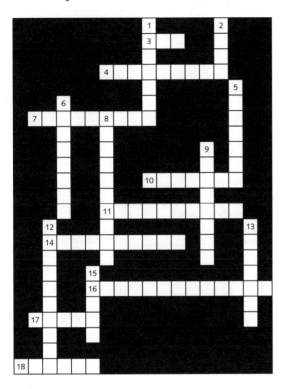

Across:

3. The main energy-transferring molecule in the body (3).
4. The basic functional unit of a skeletal muscle (9).
7. Outermost layer of connective tissue that encircles the whole muscle (9).
10. Sugar that is a major energy source for muscles (7).
11. The connective tissue that surrounds each individual muscle fiber within a fascicle (10).
14. A function of the muscular system (10).
16. The generation of heat in the body (13).
17. A protein found in thin muscle filaments (5).

18. The compound, necessary for muscular contraction, that can be stored in the muscles as myoglobin or stored in the blood as hemoglobin (6).

Down:

1. Mineral necessary for muscle contraction to occur (7).
2. The term used to describe the partial contraction of a resting muscle (4).
5. If a muscle is overstimulated it can become weak and no longer respond to stimulus. This is called muscle _____ (7).
6. Another name for smooth muscle (8).
8. The plasma membrane of a muscle cell (10).
9. Another term for a muscle cell or muscle fiber (8).
12. The ability of muscles to return to their original shape after contracting or extending (10).
13. The type of muscle that forms most of the heart (7).
15. A lack of muscle tone (5).

2. Are the following statements true or false? Write T or F in the spaces provided.

a. Smooth muscle is non-striated, involuntary, and pumps blood. _____

b. Cardiac muscle is striated and involuntary. _____

c. Skeletal muscle maintains posture and generates heat. _____

d. Skeletal muscle forms the walls of hollow internal structures such as the gastrointestinal tract. _____

e. Fascia, epimysium, perimysium, and endomysium are all types of connective tissue. _____

f. Another term for "muscle cell" is "myofilament." _____

g. Muscles contract through what is known as the sliding-filament mechanism. _____

h. Sarcomeres contain filaments that move to overlap one another and cause a muscle to shorten. _____

i. Skeletal muscles are described as striated because they are made up of bands of thick and thin filaments that appear as light and dark striations. _____

j. Thick filaments contain molecules of the proteins actin and titin. _____

3. **Fill in the missing words.**

a. There are two types of muscular contraction, _____ and _____. In an _____ contraction, muscles shorten and create movement, while the tension in the muscle remains constant. In an _____ contraction, muscles contract but do not shorten and no movement is generated.

b. _____ contractions improve strength and joint mobility, while _____ contractions stabilize joints and improve muscle tone.

c. The difference between aerobic and anaerobic processes is that aerobic processes require the presence of _____.

4. **There are three different types of skeletal muscle fibers—slow oxidative, fast oxidative, and fast glycolytic. Complete the table below.**

Features	Slow Oxidative	Fast Oxidative	Fast Glycolytic
Color	Red	Red to pink	a.
Diameter	b.	Medium	Largest
Activities	Maintains posture	c.	Fast movements such as ball throwing

5. **The figure below shows the relationship of skeletal muscles to bones. Put the following labels in their correct place:**

   1. Belly, 2. attachment/insertion, 3. fascia, 4. origin, 5. tendon

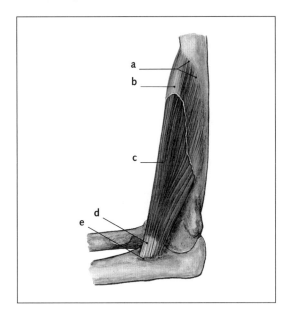

6. **Listed below are descriptions of some of the muscles of the face, scalp, and neck. Name each muscle described.**

   a. Found at the base of the skull and pulls the scalp backward when raising the eyebrows or wrinkling the forehead. _____

   b. Circles the eye and is responsible for closing it. _____

   c. Circles the mouth and moves the lips during speech. _____

   d. Moves the cheeks when sucking or blowing. _____

   e. Originates in the mandible, inserts into the chin, and is responsible for pulling up the chin or wrinkling it.

   _____

   f. Shaped like a strap and plays an important role in moving the head. It originates in the sternum and clavicle and inserts in the mastoid process.

   _____

7. **In the list below, circle only the muscles that are located on the anterior thorax and abdomen.**

   • Erector spinae

   • Serratus anterior

   • Rectus abdominis

   • Pectoralis minor

   • Trapezius

   • Infraspinatus

   • Rhomboid major

   • Splenius capitis

   • Pectoralis major

8. **Below are some of the muscles of the body. Connect the muscle to the area to which it belongs.**

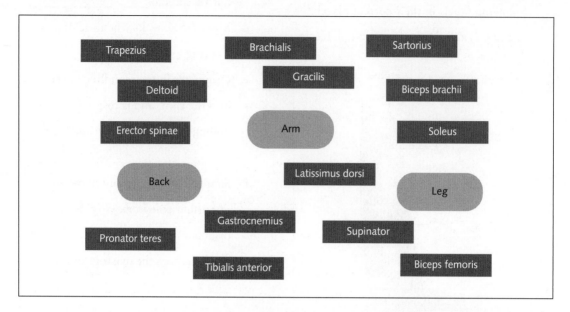

9. **In the table below, match the correct action to each muscle. Write your answers in the spaces provided.**

Term	Description
1. Soleus	**a.** Flexes middle phalanges of each finger
2. Extensor carpi ulnaris	**b.** Dorsiflexes and inverts foot and extends big toe
3. Tibialis anterior	**c.** Plantar flexes and everts the foot
4. Extensor hallucis longus	**d.** Abducts the thumb
5. Abductor pollicis brevis	**e.** Plantar flexes the foot
6. Fibularis longus	**f.** Extends and adducts the wrist
7. Flexor digitorum superficialis	**g.** Dorsiflexes the foot

Answers:

1. _____   2. _____   3. _____   4. _____   5. _____   6. _____   7. _____

Common pathologies of the muscular system

Red flags

10. **For each scenario given below state whether or not the client should be referred to a medical doctor for further examination.**
    a. Client is a 12-year-old boy whose parents bring him to you because he is losing weight, becoming progressively weaker, and losing movement in his legs.
    b. Client is an overweight 73-year-old woman with joint pain in both her knees. This pain has been coming on slowly over the past year and is worse in cold weather.
    c. Client is an overweight 73-year-old woman with joint pain in her right knee only. The knee is swollen, distinctly red, and warm to the touch. You notice that the client looks pale and is sweating and feverish.
    d. Client is a 22-year-old man who hurt his right knee when playing football last night. The knee is swollen and red, and he shrieks from pain when you gently press it.

11. **Are the following statements true or false? Write T or F in the spaces provided.**

    a. An involuntary muscle contraction is called a spasm. _____

    b. Poliomyelitis is a fungal infection. _____

    c. Fibromyalgia is characterized by aching stiffness and pain in the soft tissue. _____

    d. Myasthenia gravis and muscular dystrophy are both types of arthritis. _____

    e. Carpal tunnel syndrome is a disorder of the foot. _____

    f. The clinical term for tennis elbow is prepatellar bursitis. _____

Vocabulary test

Complete the table below.

WORD	DEFINITION
a.	A flat, sheet-like tendon that attaches muscles to bone, skin, or another muscle
b.	The wasting away of muscles
c.	Connective tissue that surrounds and protects organs, lines walls of the body, holds muscles together, and separates muscles
d.	The replacement of connective tissue by scar tissue
e.	An increase in muscle tone
f.	The point where a muscle attaches to the moving bone of a joint
g.	The point where a muscle attaches to the stationary bone of a joint
h.	A strong cord of dense connective tissue that attaches muscles to bones, to the skin, or to other muscles
i.	Muscle tissue inflammation
j.	Abnormal, involuntary muscular contraction
k.	Muscular pain
l.	Pain, stiffness, and inflammation in the joints and/or muscles
m.	Process by which muscles break down glucose
n.	Muscle tissue disease
o.	Pain in the muscles and joints of the lower back
p.	The ability of muscles to extend and lengthen

Multiple-Choice Questions

1. Which of the following is a function of the muscular system?
   a. Excretion
   b. Thermogenesis
   c. Ingestion
   d. Metabolism

2. Which type of muscle tissue contracts to help return venous blood to the heart, move lymph through the lymphatic vessels, maintain posture, and generate heat?
   a. Smooth
   b. Skeletal
   c. Cardiac
   d. Visceral

3. What types of filaments do sarcomeres contain?
   a. Thin, thick, and elastic
   b. Short, long, and wide
   c. Black, white, and red
   d. Red, white, and pink

4. Which mineral is necessary for muscle contraction to occur?
   a. Carbon dioxide
   b. Zinc
   c. Oxygen
   d. Calcium

5. Which type of muscle fibers are white, large, have a poor oxygen supply, produce ATP anaerobically, and are plentiful in muscles used for fast movements such as throwing a ball?
   a. Slow oxidative
   b. Fast oxidative
   c. Slow glycolytic
   d. Fast glycolytic

6. Which of the following statements is true?
   a. When muscles contract they shorten and usually move the moving bone toward the stationary bone
   b. The prime mover muscle always opposes the antagonist
   c. Fixators oppose the movements of both prime movers and antagonists
   d. Another term for prime mover is antagonist

7. Which of the following is not a muscle of facial expression?
   a. Occipitalis
   b. Nasalis
   c. Serratus anterior
   d. Procerus

8. Which muscle originates in the temporal and frontal bones, inserts into the mandible, and helps to move the mandible?
   a. Buccinator
   b. Risorius
   c. Sternocleidomastoid
   d. Temporalis

9. What muscle forms the floor of the thoracic cavity and functions in inhalation?
   a. Internal intercostals
   b. Diaphragm
   c. Levator scapulae
   d. Transversus abdominis

10. What is the main function of the rotator cuff muscles?
    a. To stabilize the abdominal muscles
    b. To stabilize the spinal column

c. To hold the head of the femur in the cavity of the ilium

d. To hold the head of the humerus in the cavity of the scapula

11. **What structure does the flexor pollicis brevis muscle move?**
    a. Neck
    b. Spinal column
    c. Thumb
    d. Big toe

12. **Which of the following is not a muscle located in the buttocks?**
    a. Soleus
    b. Gluteus maximus
    c. Gluteus medius
    d. Gluteus minimus

13. **What is the correct term used to describe the tearing of muscle fascia?**
    a. Sprain
    b. Strain
    c. Cramp
    d. Rupture

14. **What is the name of the cellular process through which glucose is split into pyruvic acid and ATP?**
    a. Hypertonia
    b. Hypotonia
    c. Glycolysis
    d. Thermogenesis

15. **What is the thenar eminence?**
    a. An area of soft tissue found on the ulnar side of the palm
    b. An area of soft tissue found on the radial side of the palm
    c. An area of soft tissue found beneath the little finger
    d. An area of soft tissue found in the center of the palm

6 The Nervous System

Review/Self–Study Notes

1. The nervous system has three main functions—sensory, integrative, and motor. For each of these functions write a short sentence to demonstrate to yourself that you understand it.

   • Sensory _____

   • Integrative _____

   • Motor _____

Organization of the nervous system

Because the nervous system is such a complex system it can be divided into many smaller systems. It is very important to know what these different systems are and how they function together as one coordinated whole.

2. In the space following draw your own spider diagram/mind map that shows how these divisions connect. The divisions are:
   • **Central nervous system (CNS):** This system is composed of the brain and spinal cord and functions in processing and integrating information.
   • **Peripheral nervous system (PNS):** This system is composed of the cranial and spinal nerves and it functions in transporting impulses between the CNS and the rest of the body.
   • **Somatic (voluntary) nervous system:** This system is a subdivision of the PNS. It allows us to control our skeletal muscles.
   • **Autonomic (involuntary) nervous system:** This system is a subdivision of the PNS. It controls all automatic processes of smooth muscle, cardiac muscle, and glands.
   • **Sympathetic nervous system:** This division falls under the autonomic nervous system. It stimulates activity.
   • **Parasympathetic nervous system:** This division falls under the autonomic nervous system and it works in opposition to the sympathetic nervous system by inhibiting activity.

Nervous tissue

3. The nervous system contains two types of cells—neuroglia and neurons. In the spaces provided write the basic function of each of these cells.

- Neuroglia _____

_____

_____

_____

- Neurons _____

_____

_____

_____

4. Neurons can be classified according to the type of information they carry and the direction in which they carry that information. Complete the table below.

Description	Afferent Neuron	Efferent Neuron
Alternative name (i.e., sensory or motor)		
Type of information carried (i.e., sensory or motor nerve impulse)		
Direction carried (i.e., from and to)		
Write a few words or a short phrase to remind you of this type of neuron. For example: Afferent = Arrive Efferent = Exit		

There is a third type of neuron, which has not been included in this table. This is an association neuron or interneuron. What is the function of this type of neuron?

_____

_____

_____

5. The diagram below shows the structure of a typical motor neuron. Color and label the diagram.

KEY: A MOTOR NEURON		
Structure	**Function/Description**	**Color**
Nucleus		
Cell body		
Dendrites		
Axon		
Schwann cells		
Myelin sheath		
Node of Ranvier		
Axon terminals		

6. How a nerve impulse is transmitted is quite a difficult concept to grasp. To double-check that you really do understand how nerves are transmitted, put yourself in the examiner's seat and write four questions asking about nerve transmission. Then put yourself back into your own seat and answer the questions.

Study tip

You may find it easier and more interesting if you do this exercise as part of a group.

Question 1: _____

Answer: _____

_____

_____

Question 2: _____

Answer: _____

_____

_____

Question 3: _____

Answer: _____

_____

_____

Question 4: _____

Answer: _____

_____

_____

7. Some axons are covered in a myelin sheath, which protects and insulates the axon. Color and label the diagram below of a myelinated axon.

KEY: A MYELINATED AXON		
Structure	Function/Description	Color
Axon		
Myelin sheath		
Schwann cell		
Neurilemma		
Node of Ranvier		
Neurofibril		

8. A nerve consists of a bundle of nerve fibers (axons) surrounded by connective tissue. Color and label the diagram below.

KEY: A NERVE		
Structure	**Function/Description**	**Color**
Epineurium		
Fasciculi		
Perineurium		
Endoneurium		
Nerve fiber (axon)		
Schwann cell		
Myelinated axon		
Blood vessels		

Study tip

....

Compare the connective tissue coverings of nerves to those of muscles.

9. Both the brain and the spinal cord are protected by connective tissue coverings called meninges. In the space provided, write a mnemonic to remind you of the location of each meninge:
   • Dura mater—outer covering

   • Arachnoid—middle covering

   • Pia mater—inner covering

   Mnemonic: _____

10. The brain and spinal cord are also bathed in a unique fluid called cerebrospinal fluid. List its functions.

    • _____

    • _____

    • _____

The brain

11. The figure opposite shows the human brain. Color in each region of the brain and next to the color key write three to five words that will remind you of the functions of that region.

Study tip

....

When choosing your colors, remember that the medulla oblongata, pons, and midbrain are all part of the brain stem.

KEY: THE BRAIN		
Structure	Function/Description	Color
Spinal cord		
Brain stem		
Medulla oblongata		
Pons		
Midbrain		
Cerebellum		
Diencephalon		
Cerebrum		

Cranial nerves

12. List the cranial nerves and write a short phrase or a few words to remind you of their functions.

I _____

II _____

III _____

IV _____

V _____

VI _____

VII _____

VIII _____

IX _____

X _____

XI _____

XII _____

Spinal cord

13. Describe the two main functions of the spinal cord.

• _____

• _____

14. List the differences between the gray matter and white matter of the nervous system.

	Gray Matter	White Matter
Structure		
Function		

15. There are 31 pairs of nerves that originate in the spinal cord and they all form part of the PNS because they connect the CNS to muscles or glands. Branches of some of these nerves form networks called plexuses that innervate specific structures of the body. Complete the table below.

Plexus	Area Innervated
Cervical	
Brachial	
Lumbar	
Sacral	

Special sense organs

16. Our eyes are one of the brain's most vital contacts with the outside world. However, many students find it difficult to study these fascinating structures because of the terminology involved. So to help you learn about the eye, make flash cards of the following terms and their definitions.

Lacrimal glands	Conjunctiva	Fibrous tunic
Cornea	Sclera	Vascular tunic
Iris	Ciliary body	Choroid
Photoreceptors	Vitreous body	Lens
Cones	Rods	Aqueous humor
Nervous tunic	Pigmented portion of nervous tunic	Neural portion of nervous tunic
Posterior cavity/vitreous chamber	Anterior cavity	

Study tip

Write the definitions in your own words. It is always easier to remember your own words than someone else's.

17. Color and label the following diagram of the eye.

KEY: THE EYE		
Structure	**Function/Description**	**Color**
Eyelid		
Conjunctiva		
Sclera		
Cornea		
Aqueous humor		
Pupil		

KEY: THE EYE		
Structure	**Function/Description**	**Color**
Iris		
Ciliary body		
Lens		
Choroid		
Retina		
Fovea		
Optic disc		
Optic nerve		
Vitreous humor		

18. Our ears enable us to hear, locate sounds, and maintain our balance. They can be divided into three regions—the external or outer ear that we see, the middle ear, and the internal or inner ear. In order to learn these different regions of the ear, draw the "journey" of a sound wave in the space provided below. The first few steps have been done for you.

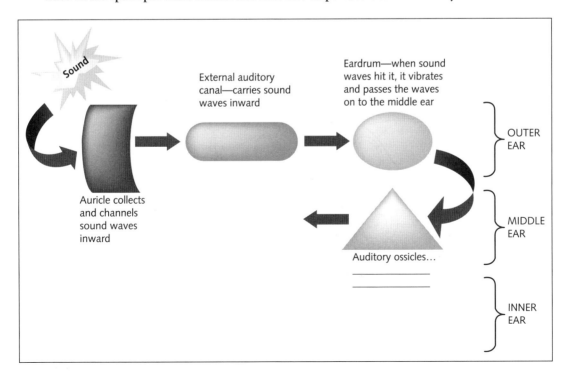

19. Now, color and label the following diagram of the ear.

KEY: THE EAR		
Structure	Function/Description	Color
External ear (auricle)		
External auditory canal (meatus)		
Tympanic membrane		
Malleus		
Incus		
Stapes		
Eustachian tube		
Semicircular canals		
Cochlea		
Temporal bone		

20. Color and label the following diagram of the mouth.

KEY: THE MOUTH		
Structure	**Function/Description**	**Color**
Lips		
Tongue		
Filiform papillae		
Fungiform papillae		
Vallate papillae		
Soft palate		
Uvula		
Palatoglossal fold		
Palatopharyngeal fold		
Palatine tonsil		

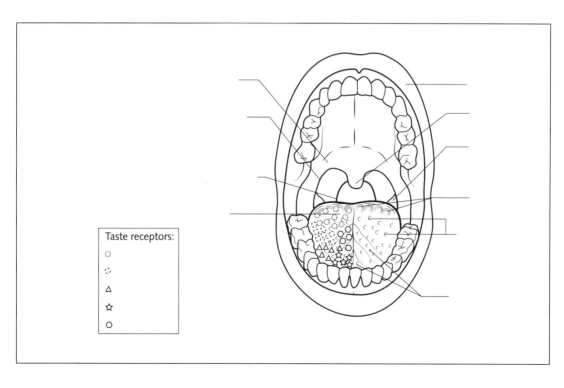

21. Color and label the following diagram of the nose.

KEY: THE NOSE		
Structure	**Function/Description**	**Color**
Nasal cavity		
Olfactory area		
Pharyngeal orifice of auditory tube		
Pharynx		
Larynx		
Palate		

22. The senses of taste and smell are closely connected because they both use the same types of receptors. These receptors are called chemoreceptors and are stimulated by chemical molecules. Bearing this in mind, create a flow diagram of the movement of a molecule of coffee from when you first smell and then taste the coffee to when your brain recognizes (and hopefully enjoys) it.

Common pathologies of the nervous system

Red flags
23. In the box below describe all the symptoms of a stroke.

24. Write down a short phrase that will remind you of each of the following diseases and disorders.

    Nervous system diseases and disorders:

    - Alzheimer's disease _____

    - Anosmia _____

    - Brain tumor _____

    - Cerebral palsy _____

    - Cerebrovascular accident (CVA, stroke)

      _____

    - Dementia _____

    - Depression _____

    - Epilepsy _____

    - Fainting (syncope) _____

    - Insomnia _____

    - Meningitis _____

    - Motor neurone disease (MND)

      _____

    - Myalgic encephalomyelitis
      (ME, chronic fatigue) _____

    - Pain and referred pain (synalgia)

      _____

    - Parkinson's disease (PD) _____

- Spina bifida _____
- Cluster headaches _____
- Migraines _____
- Spinal cord injuries _____
- Transient ischemic attack _____
- Tension headaches _____

Nerve disorders:

- Bell's palsy _____
- Multiple sclerosis _____
- Neuritis _____
- Trigeminal neuralgia _____

Head injuries:

- Concussion _____
- Contusion _____
- Laceration _____

Eye disorders:

- Cataract _____
- Conjunctivitis (pink eye) _____
- Corneal ulcer _____
- Glaucoma _____
- Stye (hordeolum) _____

Ear disorders:

- Deafness _____
- Earache _____
- Glue ear (secretory or serous

  otitis media) _____
- Otitis media _____
- Tinnitus _____
- Vertigo _____

Exercises

1. The nervous system can be divided into the central nervous system (CNS) and peripheral nervous system (PNS). Complete the spider diagram below, using arrows to connect the structures and functions to where they belong, either the CNS or PNS.

2. The peripheral nervous system can also be split into subdivisions. Complete the diagram below by filling in the missing words on the lines provided.

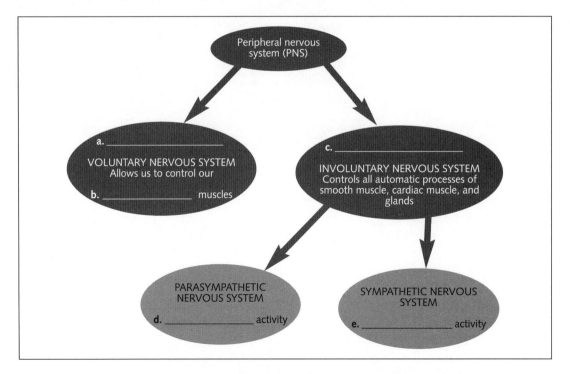

3. **Are the following statements true or false? Write T or F in the spaces provided.**

   a. Afferent neurons conduct impulses from sensory receptors to the CNS.

   _____

   b. Motor neurons are also called afferent neurons. _____

   c. The sympathetic nervous system decreases the heartbeat. _____

   d. The parasympathetic nervous system opposes the actions of the sympathetic nervous system by inhibiting activity and conserving energy. _____

   e. Neuroglia are the cells responsible for maintaining the homeostasis of the fluid surrounding neurons. _____

   f. Efferent neurons transmit information from the skin, sense organs, muscles, joints, and viscera to the CNS. _____

4. **All neurons have three parts—a cell body, dendrites, and an axon terminal. Complete this table on the structure of a typical motor neuron.**

Structure	Function
a.	The metabolic center of a neuron
Dendrite	b.
Axon	c.
d.	Chemical that influences other neurons, muscle fibers, or gland cells
e.	Neurotransmitter-containing sac found at the end of axons
Myelin sheath	f.
g.	Cells that form the myelin sheath
Nodes of Ranvier (neurofibril nodes)	h.

5. The figure below is an overview of the brain. Complete the labeling.

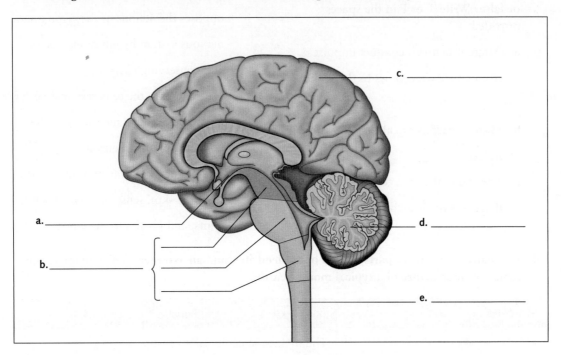

6. Use the clues given to unscramble the letters below. Write your answers in the spaces provided.

a. RDUAAETMR _____

b. EICNVTESLR _____

c. EMINESNG _____

d. RAHDAOCNI _____

Clues:
- These three layers cover the brain and help protect it from the external environment
- The outer connective tissue covering of the brain
- The middle connective tissue covering of the brain
- Cavities in the brain through which CSF can flow

7. Use the clues below to complete this word search.

L	I	M	B	I	C	S	Y	S	T	E	M	D	F	H	C
D	G	J	T	X	A	D	W	I	G	E	I	G	A	F	E
S	D	G	W	C	E	R	E	B	R	U	M	C	N	A	R
D	D	L	E	E	O	D	T	G	I	O	D	E	S	E	E
E	O	Q	B	R	A	I	N	S	T	E	M	O	W	D	B
P	Y	F	O	E	H	E	D	H	W	P	K	H	T	H	R
H	R	J	T	B	D	N	O	D	E	D	G	V	E	O	A
Y	H	F	F	E	J	C	T	U	L	E	S	A	U	I	L
F	V	C	A	L	D	E	G	I	V	U	N	F	T	G	C
K	M	O	W	L	X	P	F	R	E	S	C	J	S	J	O
V	V	A	G	U	S	H	A	P	Q	U	W	D	T	N	R
E	B	T	X	M	X	A	B	D	U	C	E	N	S	E	T
J	Y	V	D	F	E	L	S	O	T	T	O	G	R	C	E
U	I	D	X	A	T	O	L	F	A	C	T	O	R	Y	X
E	R	J	D	D	R	N	G	S	F	G	T	A	G	B	I

Clues (note, these are not in order):
- It connects the spinal cord to the diencephalon.
- The area of the brain responsible for movement, posture, and balance. It is found at the back of the head.

- It houses the pituitary and pineal endocrine glands, and also contains the epithalamus, thalamus, and hypothalamus. It is sometimes called the interbrain. It is the area of the brain that gives us the ability to read, write, speak, remember, create, and imagine. It is often referred to as the "seat of intelligence."
- The "emotional brain": the area of the brain associated with pain and pleasure as well as memory.
- The cerebrum's outermost layer. It is made up of gray matter.
- How many pairs of cranial nerves are there?
- Cranial nerve I: this nerve functions in the sense of smell.
- Cranial nerve VI: this nerve helps control the movement of the eyeball.
- Cranial nerve X: this nerve helps control the secretion of digestive fluids and the contraction and relaxation of the smooth muscle of the organs of the thoracic and abdominal cavities.

8. **As part of the CNS, the spinal cord is integral to maintaining the homeostasis of the body. In the table below, match the structures to the functions and write your answers in the spaces provided.**

Structure	Function
1. White matter	**a.** A network of nerves
2. Cauda equina	**b.** Neurological tissue that contains myelinated neurons and functions in transporting impulses
3. Gray matter	**c.** The thin, inner connective tissue covering of the spinal cord
4. Plexus	**d.** A bundle-like structure of nerves that extends from the end of the spinal cord
5. Pia mater	**e.** Neurological tissue that contains unmyelinated neurons and functions in receiving and integrating information

Answers:

1. _____   2. _____   3. _____   4. _____   5. _____

9. **The figure opposite shows the structure of the eyeball. Label the following areas:**

1. Iris   2. Cornea   3. Lens   4. Anterior cavity

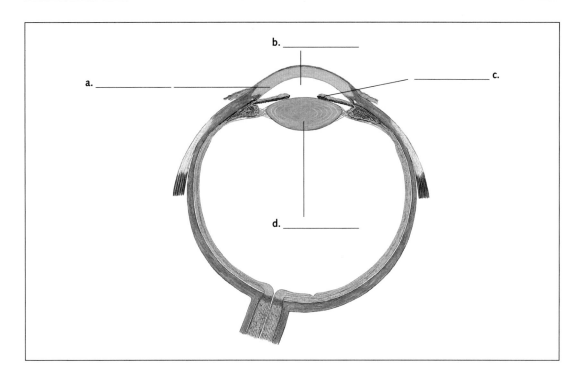

a. _____ _____
b. _____
c. _____
d. _____

10. **Fill in the missing words.**

   a. The _____ ear collects and channels sound waves inward. The part of
      the ear that we see is called the _____. The eardrum is also called the
      _____ membrane, and when sound waves hit it, it _____,
      passing the waves on to the _____ ear.

   b. The _____ ear is a small air-filled cavity that is partitioned from the outer
      ear by the _____ and from the inner ear by the _____ window
      and the _____ window. The middle ear contains three tiny bones, the
      _____, _____, and _____. Together these bones are called the
      _____ _____. The middle ear is connected to the throat by the
      _____ _____.

   c. The _____ ear is sometimes also called the labyrinth, and it consists of a
      bony labyrinth filled with a fluid called _____, enclosing a membranous
      labyrinth filled with a fluid called _____. The labyrinth is divided into three
      areas—the _____, the three semicircular _____, and the organ of
      _____.

11. **Are the following statements true or false? Write T or F in the spaces provided.**

   a. The receptors of taste are called gustatory receptors and they are found in taste buds on the tongue, on the back of the roof of the mouth, and in the pharynx and larynx. _____

   b. Gustatory receptor cells are also called Bowman's glands. _____

   c. Gustatory receptor cells are chemoreceptors. _____

   d. The receptors of smell are called olfactory receptors. _____

   e. The senses of taste and smell are linked, and their impulses travel to the cerebellum in the brain. _____

Common pathologies of the nervous system

12. **Give the names of the following pathologies of the nervous system.**

   a. Inflammation of the meninges that cover the brain and spinal cord _____

   b. Disorders of the brain characterized by seizures that are short, recurrent, periodic attacks of motor, sensory, or psychological malfunction _____

   c. The loss of the sense of smell _____

   d. The progressive degeneration of brain tissue; symptoms include memory loss, forgetfulness, disorientation, and confusion _____

   e. A birth defect in which the spinal vertebrae do not form normally _____

   f. Weakness or paralysis of the muscles on one side of the face _____

   g. The inflammation of a nerve or a group of nerves _____

   h. Inflammation of the sciatic nerve _____

   i. The temporary loss of consciousness following a head injury _____

   j. Loss of vision due to abnormally high pressure in the eye; a result of the eye's inability to drain aqueous humor as quickly as it produces it _____

Vocabulary test

Complete the table below.

WORD	DEFINITION
a. _____	A bundle or knot of nerve cell bodies
b. _____	The three connective tissue membranes that enclose the brain and spinal cord

WORD	DEFINITION
c. _____	The study of the nervous system
d. _____	A specialized nerve receptor located in muscles, joints, and tendons that provides sensory information regarding body position and movements
e. _____	The ability to transmit an impulse from a neuron to another neuron, muscle, or gland
f. _____	Area of the brain that regulates homeostasis and relays sensory impulses to the cerebral cortex
g. _____	A clear, colorless liquid that surrounds the CNS, protecting it and helping it to maintain homeostasis
h. _____	An electrically charged molecule
i. _____	The ability to respond to a stimulus and convert it into an impulse
j. _____	The organs of the abdominal body cavity

Multiple-Choice Questions

1. The part of the nervous system that reacts to changes by stimulating activity is called the:
   a. Somatic nervous system
   b. Autonomic nervous system
   c. Sympathetic nervous system
   d. Parasympathetic nervous system

2. How many different types of cells does the nervous system contain?
   a. One
   b. Two
   c. Three
   d. Four

3. What type of neuron transmits impulses from the skin to the CNS?
   a. Afferent
   b. Efferent

   c. Association
   d. Interneuron

4. What type of neuron transmits impulses from the CNS to muscles?
   a. Afferent
   b. Efferent
   c. Association
   d. Interneuron

5. What is another name for afferent neurons?
   a. Sensory neurons
   b. Motor neurons
   c. Mixed neurons
   d. Interneurons

6. Where on a motor neuron are the synaptic vesicles found?
   a. In the myelin sheath
   b. At the end of the dendrites
   c. At the end of the cell body
   d. At the end of the axons

7. How are nerve impulses transmitted?
   a. Electronically
   b. Chemically
   c. Electrochemically
   d. None of the above

8. What are the two ions necessary for the transmission of a nerve impulse?
   a. Sodium and potassium
   b. Calcium and magnesium
   c. Potassium and calcium
   d. Magnesium and sodium

9. Which of the following statements is true?
   a. The three meninges are the outer pia mater, the middle arachnoid, and the inner dura mater
   b. The brain stem consists of the medulla oblongata, cerebellum, and diencephalon
   c. The cerebrum consists of the cerebral cortex, which is the white matter of the brain
   d. The brain is protected by the bones of the cranium, the meninges, and cerebrospinal fluid

10. Which of the following is not a region of the brain?
    a. Brain stem
    b. Diencephalon
    c. Pineal
    d. Cerebrum

11. Which of the following are all cranial nerves?
    a. Optic, trigeminal, facial, accessory
    b. Olfactory, brachial, abducens, trochlear

c. Hypoglossal, cervical, lumbar, vagus
d. Thoracic, oculomotor, vestibulocochlear, glossopharyngeal

12. Approximately where in the spinal column does the spinal cord end?
    a. C3
    b. T2
    c. L2
    d. S3

13. How many pairs of spinal nerves are there?
    a. 11
    b. 21
    c. 31
    d. 41

14. Which of the following areas of the body is not served by the lumbar plexus?
    a. Abdominal wall
    b. Buttocks
    c. External genitals
    d. Lower limb

15. Which of the following statements is true?
    a. Light waves are bent as they pass through the structures of the eyeball; they then hit the retina where they are converted into nerve impulses
    b. Sound waves are transmitted as vibrations through the outer ear until they reach the middle ear where they are converted into nerve impulses
    c. Tastes are chemicals that come into contact with hairlike projections on olfactory receptors where they are converted into nerve impulses
    d. Smells are chemicals that dissolve in mucus in the nose; they then come into contact with taste buds and are converted into nerve impulses

7 The Endocrine System

Review/Self–Study Notes

Functions of the endocrine system

1. There are two types of glands in the body—endocrine and exocrine. Complete the table below to highlight the differences between these glands.

	Endocrine Gland	Exocrine Gland
Where are substances secreted?		
What happens to the secretions?		
Examples of secretions:		
Write a few words or a short phrase to remind you of each type of gland		

2. Hormone secretion is controlled by signals from the nervous system (neural stimulation), chemical changes in the blood, and other hormones. Describe each of these in your own words.

- Neural stimulation _____

  _____

- Chemical changes _____

  _____

- Hormonal stimulation _____

  _____

The endocrine glands and their hormones

3. The endocrine system is another of those systems in which you will find a great deal of information that you simply have to remember. Once again, the only way to really do this is to sit down and memorize it all. To help you do this, firstly complete the following table and then make flash cards of the information contained in the table.

Study tip

Write the actions in your own words, or sketch pictures if you find it easier to remember images rather than words.

Gland	Hormone	Action
Anterior pituitary	Human growth hormone	
	Thyroid-stimulating hormone	
	Follicle-stimulating hormone	
	Luteinizing hormone	
	Prolactin	
	Adrenocorticotropic hormone	
	Melanocyte-stimulating hormone	
Posterior pituitary	Oxytocin	
	Antidiuretic hormone (vasopressin)	
Pineal	Melatonin	
Thyroid	Thyroid hormone	
	Calcitonin	

Gland	Hormone	Action
Parathyroids	Parathormone	
Thymus	Thymosin	
Pancreatic islets	Glucagon	
	Insulin	
	Somatostatin	
Adrenal cortex	Mineralocorticoids	
	Glucocorticoids	
	Sex hormones	
Adrenal medulla	Epinephrine (adrenaline)	
	Norepinephrine (noradrenaline)	
Ovaries	Estrogens	
	Progesterone	
Testes	Testosterone	

Study group

To help you revise your knowledge of the endocrine system, use the flash cards you have just made and play the game "30 seconds" (see chapter 1 to learn how to play).

4. Color and label the endocrine glands in the diagram below.

KEY: THE ENDOCRINE GLANDS			
Gland	Color	Gland	Color
Hypothalamus		Thymus	
Pituitary		Adrenals	
Pineal		Pancreatic islets	
Thyroid		Ovaries (in a female)	
Parathyroids		Testes (in a male)	

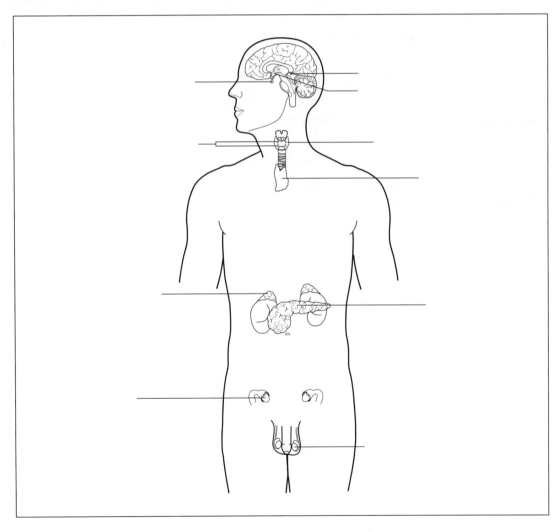

5. Listed below are both general effects and red flags associated with hormonal disorders. Take time to think about why these signs and symptoms are occurring and write your answers in the table. Think about which hormones or glands are involved and what could possibly be causing the problem. What can go wrong if the problem is not rectified? Take note that there may be a few different explanations for each sign or symptom.

Sign or Symptom	Possible Causes/Explanations
Severe headaches	
Failure to thrive (lethargy, depression, weight loss, weakness)	
Weight gain	
Changes in heat tolerance	
Increased urination and increased thirst	
Palpitations	
Sweating	
Coarsening of features	

Sign or Symptom	Possible Causes/Explanations
Delayed puberty	
Virilization or hirsutism	

Common pathologies of the endocrine system

6. Write down a short phrase that will remind you of each of the following diseases and disorders.

Pathologies of the adrenal glands:

- Addison's disease _____
- Cushing's syndrome _____

Pathologies of the pancreatic islets:

- Diabetes mellitus _____

Pathologies of the parathyroid glands:

- Hypocalcemia (calcium deficiency) _____

Pathologies of the pineal gland:

- Seasonal affective disorder (SAD) _____

Pathologies of the pituitary gland:

- Acromegaly _____
- Diabetes insipidus _____
- Gigantism _____

Pathologies of the thyroid gland:

- Goiter _____
- Graves' disease _____
- Hashimoto's disease _____
- Myxedema (hypothyroidism) _____
- Thyrotoxicosis (hyperthyroidism) _____

Exercises

1. Are the following statements true or false? Write T or F in the spaces provided.

   a. Hormones are chemical messengers that are secreted by exocrine glands. _____

   b. Hormones coordinate body functions such as growth, development, reproduction, metabolism, and homeostasis. _____

   c. Hormones such as insulin and oxytocin are steroid hormones. _____

   d. Hormone secretion is controlled by signals from the nervous system, chemical changes in the blood, and other hormones. _____

   e. One of the key differences between the nervous and endocrine systems is that the nervous system takes longer to act than the endocrine system does. _____

   f. The time at which a child becomes sexually mature is called the menopause. _____

2. The columns below show the major endocrine glands and the hormones they secrete. However, some of these hormones are in the wrong columns. Cross out the hormones that are in the incorrect columns and write their names in the correct columns.

PITUITARY	PINEAL	THYROID	PARATHYROIDS	THYMUS
Human growth hormone	Prolactin	Thyroid hormone	Parathormone	Adrenocortico-tropic hormone
Glucagon	Epinephrine (adrenaline)	Thymosin	Melatonin	Sex hormones
Calcitonin		Thyroid-stimulating hormone		

PANCREAS	ADRENAL CORTEX	ADRENAL MEDULLA	OVARIES	TESTES
Antidiuretic hormone (vasopressin)	Mineralocorticoids	Follicle-stimulating hormone	Estrogens	Luteinizing hormone
Somatostatin	Norephinephrine (noradrenaline)	Testosterone	Oxytocin	Progesterone
	Glucocorticoids	Insulin	Melanocyte-stimulating hormone	

3. **Complete the crossword below.**

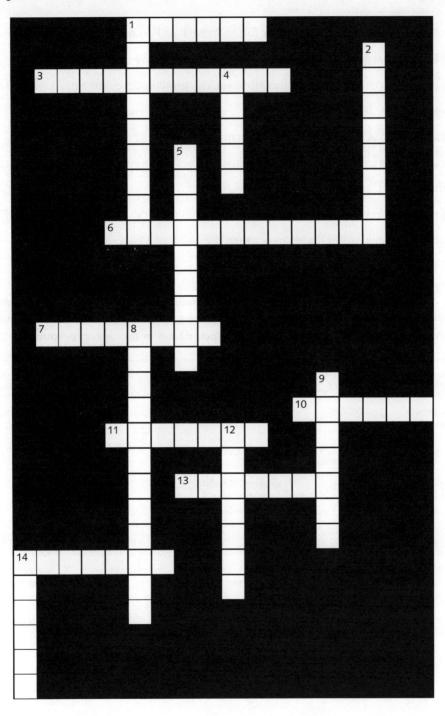

Across:

1. This endocrine gland secretes a hormone that is thought to contribute to setting the timing of the body's biological clock (6).
3. This gland releases a hormone that helps control blood calcium levels (11).
6. An endocrine gland that is also considered part of the nervous system (12).
7. A gland that secretes substances into ducts, which then carry these substances into body cavities or to the outer surface of the body (8).
10. The male sex glands (6).
11. A chemical messenger that is transported by the blood and that regulates cellular activity (7).
13. These two glands are found above the kidneys (7).
14. This butterfly-shaped gland is found wrapped around the trachea, just below the larynx (7).

Down:

1. The endocrine gland that secretes human growth hormone, luteinizing hormone, and adrenocorticotropic hormone, amongst other hormones (9).
2. This structure functions as part of both the digestive and endocrine systems, and its endocrine function is to help regulate blood glucose levels (8).
4. A female sex gland (5).
5. A hormone-secreting gland (9).
8. A body function controlled and coordinated by hormones (12).

9. The region of the adrenal glands that releases hormones that function in the fight-or-flight response of the body and help the body cope with stress (7).
12. A body system that works closely with the endocrine system to control all the processes that take place in the body (7).
14. This gland is located in the thorax, behind the sternum and between the lungs (6).

Common pathologies of the endocrine system

4. **Fill in the missing words.**

   a. Addison's disease is caused by

      _____ of glucocorticoids and aldosterone.

   b. _____ _____

      is a disorder in which there is an

      elevation of glucose in the blood.

      Signs and symptoms include increased

      thirst and urination.

   c. Hypocalcemia is a deficiency of the

      mineral _____.

   d. The letters SAD stand for

      _____ _____

      _____, which is

      characterized by depression, a lack

      of interest in one's usual activities,

      oversleeping, and overeating.

e. Hypersecretion of human growth hormone can cause _____ in adults or _____ in children.

f. Diabetes insipidus is caused by a lack of _____ hormone.

g. An enlarged thyroid gland is called a _____.

h. Myxedema is also called _____ and is caused by the hyposecretion of thyroid hormones in adults.

i. _____ disease is a hereditary autoimmune disorder in which the thyroid gland is continually stimulated to produce hormones.

j. Hashimoto's disease is a disorder of the _____ gland.

Vocabulary test

Complete the table below.

WORD	DEFINITION
Apoptosis	a.
Endocrinology	b.
Gonads	c.
Hypersecretion	d.
Hyposecretion	e.
f.	The development of male physical characteristics
g.	An enlarged thyroid gland
h.	The day/night (24 hour) cycle of the body
i.	Group of hormones responsible for the flight-or-flight response

Multiple-Choice Questions

1. Which of the following is not a characteristic of a hormone?
   a. Chemical messenger
   b. Secreted by exocrine glands
   c. Transported in the blood
   d. Regulates cellular activity

2. Steroid hormones include:
   a. Sex hormones
   b. Insulin
   c. Oxytocin
   d. Amino-acid-based hormones

3. Which of the following statements is correct?
   a. Hormones are transported along nerve axons
   b. Hormones generally act more quickly than nerve impulses
   c. Hormones only affect muscle cells
   d. Hormones help coordinate metabolic activities, growth, development, and reproduction

4. Which gland does the hypothalamus have its greatest influence on?
   a. Pituitary
   b. Pineal
   c. Thyroid
   d. Thymus

5. Where in the body is the pituitary gland located?
   a. In the head, at the base of the occipital lobe
   b. In the head, behind the nose and between the eyes
   c. In the throat, below the larynx
   d. In the chest, between the lungs

6. Which of the following are all hormones secreted by the pituitary gland?
   a. Follicle-stimulating hormone, estrogen, melatonin
   b. Epinephrine, antidiuretic hormone (vasopressin), parathormone
   c. Human growth hormone, oxytocin, prolactin
   d. Calcitonin, luteinizing hormone, melanocyte-stimulating hormone

7. What is the main action of oxytocin?
   a. Stimulates the development of oocytes
   b. Stimulates ovulation
   c. Stimulates contraction of the uterus during labor
   d. Has an antidiuretic effect

8. Which hormone increases blood pressure, dilates airways to the lungs, decreases the rate of digestion, and increases blood glucose levels?
   a. Insulin
   b. Progesterone
   c. Parathormone
   d. Epinephrine

9. Which hormone does the pineal gland secrete?
   a. Thymosin
   b. Melatonin
   c. Melanocyte-stimulating hormone
   d. Calcitonin

10. Which hormone is responsible for the development of masculine secondary sex characteristics?
    a. Testosterone
    b. Estrogen
    c. Progesterone
    d. Somatostatin

11. **What is menopause characterized by?**
    a. The appearance of secondary sexual characteristics
    b. The start of menstruation
    c. The cessation of ovulation and menstruation
    d. The development of a fetus

12. **The hormone calcitonin is secreted by which endocrine gland?**
    a. Thyroid
    b. Parathyroid
    c. Thymus
    d. Pancreas

13. **Adrenocorticotropic hormone is secreted by which endocrine gland?**
    a. Adrenals
    b. Pineal
    c. Pituitary
    d. Pancreas

14. **Which of the following best describes glucocorticoids?**
    a. A group of hormones that regulate the mineral content of the blood
    b. A group of hormones that regulate metabolism and help the body resist long-term stressors
    c. A group of hormones that function in the body's fight-or-flight response
    d. A group of hormones that slow absorption of nutrients from the gastrointestinal tract

15. **Which of the following are all signs and symptoms of Cushing's syndrome?**
    a. Increased thirst and urination, weight loss, fatigue, and blurred vision
    b. Confusion, memory loss, depression, muscle aches and spasms
    c. The abnormal lengthening of the long bones of the arms and legs
    d. Fatigue and excessive fat deposits on the face, torso, and back

8 The Respiratory System

Review/Self–Study Notes

Structure and functions of the respiratory system

1. The primary function of the respiratory system is respiration, which is the exchange of gases. Complete the table below, which highlights the differences between the various types of respiration.

	Pulmonary Ventilation	External Respiration	Internal Respiration	Cellular/ Respiration Oxidation
Description	This is another term for breathing, which includes both inspiration and expiration			This is a metabolic reaction in which oxygen is used and carbon dioxide is formed as a by-product
Where does this occur?	Lungs	Between lungs and blood	Between blood and tissue cells	In cells
Is oxygen gained or lost?	On inspiration oxygen is gained and on expiration oxygen is lost			
Is carbon dioxide gained or lost?				
Write a few words or a short phrase to remind you of this process				

The respiratory system takes in oxygen from the air we breathe, and this air travels through a series of interconnecting passageways from the nose to the alveoli where gaseous exchange between the lungs and blood finally takes place.

2. In order to learn the structures of the respiratory system, draw the journey of air in the space provided. As you label each structure, write down any important information that you will need to remember (for example, structure and function). The first step in this journey has been done for you.

Nose
Air breathed in through external nares (nostrils) is filtered, warmed, and moistened. Nose also receives olfactory stimuli and acts as a resonating chamber for sound.

3. **The lungs are an unusual organ in that they have two blood supplies:**
    *   Pulmonary arteries bring deoxygenated blood to the lungs. Here the blood is oxygenated by the lungs, and this oxygenated blood is then transported to the heart by the pulmonary veins.
    *   Bronchial arteries bring oxygenated blood to the lung tissue. Most of this blood is returned to the heart by the pulmonary veins; however, some of it drains into bronchial veins, which then transport the blood to the heart via the superior vena cava.

    In the space provided below, draw a spider diagram or mind map of the above information.

4. Color and label the following diagrams of the respiratory system, lungs, and alveolus.

KEY: THE RESPIRATORY SYSTEM		
Structure	Function/Description	Color
Nasal cavity		
Pharynx		
Epiglottis		
Larynx		
Esophagus		
Trachea		
Right lung		
Left lung		
Bronchus		
Bronchioles		
Pleural cavity		
Pleural membranes		
Ribs		
Intercostal muscles		
Diaphragm		

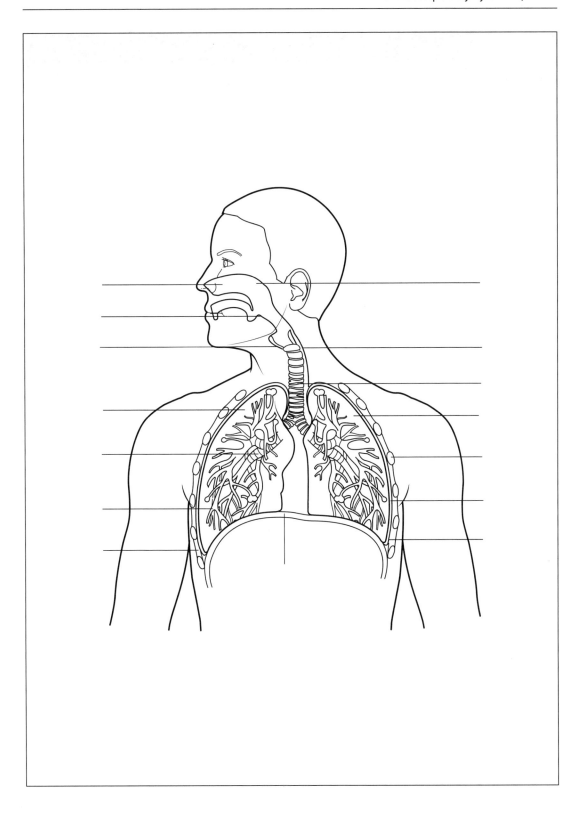

KEY: THE LUNGS		
Structure	Function/Description	Color
Right lung	Number of lobes:	
Left lung	Number of lobes:	
Trachea		
Carina		
Right main bronchus		
Left main bronchus		
Lobar bronchi		
Segmental bronchi		

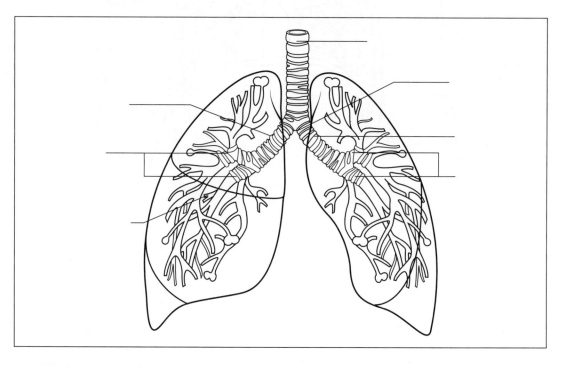

KEY: THE ALVEOLUS		
Structure	**Function/Description**	**Color**
Bronchiole		
Alveolus		
Capillary from pulmonary artery	Do these carry oxygenated or deoxygenated blood?	
Capillary to pulmonary vein	Do these carry oxygenated or deoxygenated blood?	
Network of capillaries surrounding alveolus		

Physiology of respiration

5. Pulmonary ventilation, or breathing, is dependent on the existence of a pressure gradient between the pressure inside the lungs and that outside them. To help you remember the physiology of respiration, make up mnemonics using the information given below. Before you do this, however, rewrite Boyle's Law in your own words to ensure you understand it.

   • Boyle's Law = The pressure of a gas in a closed container is inversely proportional to the volume of the container.

   Rewrite this law in your own words: _____

   _____

   _____

   • Inspiration: diaphragm and external intercostal muscles contract—this causes the thoracic cavity to increase in size, which causes the pressure inside the thoracic cavity to drop, creating a vacuum that sucks air inward.

   Mnemonic: _____

   • Normal expiration (a passive process): muscles recoil to their natural size—this causes the thoracic cavity to decrease in size, therefore the atmospheric pressure is less than the pressure within the lungs, thus air moves out of the lungs.

   Mnemonic: _____

   • Active expiration: abdominal and internal intercostal muscles contract—this forces the diaphragm upward, which reduces the size of the thoracic cavity and thereby reduces the volume of the lungs, increasing the pressure within the lungs; therefore, air is forced out of the lungs.

   Mnemonic: _____

6. External respiration (pulmonary respiration) is the exchange of oxygen and carbon dioxide between the alveoli and blood. In your own words, summarize this process.

   _____

   _____

   _____

   _____

7. Color and label the following diagram showing gaseous exchange between the alveoli and capillaries.

KEY: GASEOUS EXCHANGE BETWEEN THE ALVEOLI AND CAPILLARIES		
Structure	Function/Description	Color
Wall of capillary		
Red blood cell		
Wall of alveolus		
Layer of moisture lining alveolus		

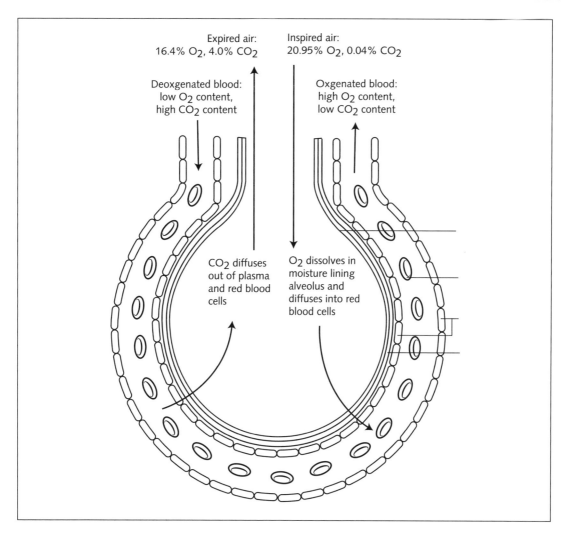

Expired air:
16.4% O_2, 4.0% CO_2

Inspired air:
20.95% O_2, 0.04% CO_2

Deoxgenated blood:
low O_2 content,
high CO_2 content

Oxgenated blood:
high O_2 content,
low CO_2 content

CO_2 diffuses
out of plasma
and red blood
cells

O_2 dissolves in
moisture lining
alveolus and
diffuses into red
blood cells

Common pathologies of the respiratory system

Red flags

8. Listed below are respiratory conditions that should always be referred to a medical doctor for further examination. Beneath each condition, write a short description of why you think this condition should be referred on.
   - Difficulty in breathing, shortness of breath or rapid breathing, especially if accompanied by accessory muscle use

     _____

   - A high-pitched wheezing sound when breathing

     _____

   - Respiratory signs and symptoms accompanied by tachycardia, bradycardia, changes in blood pressure, confusion, sweating, pallor, anxiety, or confusion

     _____

   - Severe chest pain or chest pain referred to the neck or shoulders

     _____

   - Coughing up of blood (hemoptysis)

     _____

   - Weight loss and night sweats

     _____

9. Write down a short phrase that will remind you of each of the following diseases and disorders.

   Chronic obstructive pulmonary disease (COPD):
   - Asthma _____

   - Status asthmaticus _____
   - Bronchitis _____
   - Emphysema _____

Infectious and environmentally related diseases and disorders:
   - Asbestosis _____
   - Bronchiolitis _____
   - Cor pulmonale _____
   - Cystic fibrosis _____
   - Hay fever _____
   - Hyperventilation _____
   - Influenza _____
   - Laryngitis _____
   - Lung cancer _____
   - Methicillin-resistant *Staphylococcus aureus* (MRSA) _____
   - Pharyngitis _____
   - Pleurisy _____
   - Pneumonia _____
   - Pneumothorax _____
   - Pulmonary embolism _____
   - Pulmonary fibrosis _____
   - Rhinitis _____
   - Sarcoidosis _____
   - Severe acute respiratory syndrome (SARS) _____
   - Sinusitis _____
   - Tuberculosis (TB) _____
   - Whooping cough (pertussis) _____

Exercises

1. The table below gives some of the terminology particular to the respiratory system. Match each term to its correct definition, and write your answers in the spaces provided.

Term	Definition
1. Pulmonary ventilation	a. The exchange of gases between the lungs and the blood
2. External respiration	b. Area formed by the alveoli where the exchange of gases occurs
3. Internal respiration	c. A series of passageways that allows air to reach the lungs—includes the nose, pharynx, larynx, trachea, and bronchi
4. Cellular respiration	d. Another term for breathing—the act in which air is breathed into and out of the lungs
5. Olfaction	e. The exchange of gases between blood and tissue cells
6. Conducting zone	f. The metabolic reaction that takes place within a cell
7. Respiratory zone	g. The sense of smell

Answers:

1. _____   2. _____   3. _____   4. _____   5. _____   6. _____   7. _____

2. The figure below shows the structures of the respiratory system. Complete the labeling of this diagram.

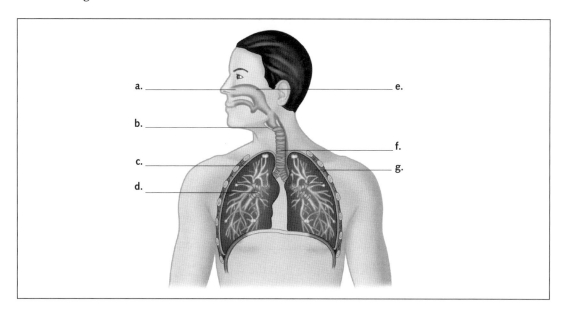

3. Match the respiratory structures to their functions and write the answers in the spaces provided below. Please note that some structures have more than one function.

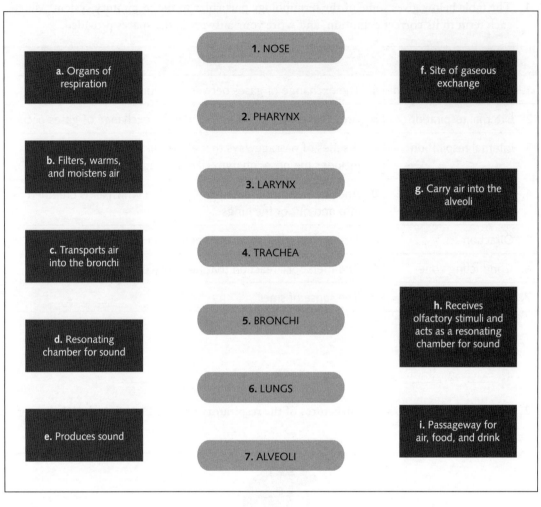

Answers:

1. _____ 2. _____ 3. _____ 4. _____ 5. _____ 6. _____ 7. _____

4. **Below is an outline of the blood supply to the lungs. Fill in the missing words.**

   a. Pulmonary _____ bring _____ blood to the lungs. _____ blood is then transported from the lungs to the heart by the pulmonary _____.

   b. _____ arteries bring oxygenated blood to the lung tissue. Most of this blood is returned to the heart by the _____ veins. However, some of it drains into the _____ veins, which transport it to the superior _____ _____ and then to the heart.

5. **Are the following statements true or false? Write T or F in the spaces provided.**

   a. Pulmonary ventilation is dependent on the existence of a pressure gradient between the pressure inside the lungs and that outside the lungs. _____

   b. Expiration is the movement of air from the atmosphere into the lungs. _____

   c. Inspiration occurs when the diaphragm and external intercostal muscles contract. _____

   d. During normal, quiet breathing, expiration is a passive process that does not involve any muscular contraction. _____

   e. In external respiration, oxygen moves from the alveolar air into the blood through the process of osmosis. _____

   f. In internal respiration, blood loses carbon dioxide and gains oxygen. _____

   g. Air is a mixture of oxygen, carbon dioxide, nitrogen, water vapor, and a small quantity of inert gases. _____

Common pathologies of the respiratory system

6. **Identify the following pathologies, and write the answers in the spaces provided.**

   a. A chronic disorder characterized by "attacks" in which a person struggles to exhale, has difficulty breathing, and wheezes and coughs. Attacks can be caused by stimuli ranging from pollen and house dust mites to cold air or emotional upsets.

   _____

   b. An irreversible disease in which the alveolar walls disintegrate, leaving abnormally large air spaces in the lungs. The main sign of this disease is the inability to exhale easily.

   _____

   c. Abnormally fast breathing when the body is at rest. Symptoms include dizziness, tingling sensations, and a tightness across the chest. _____

   d. Inflammation of the larynx. Characterized by hoarseness or voice loss, a sore throat, and a painful or tickling cough. _____

   e. Inflammation of the mucous membrane lining the nose. Signs and symptoms include a runny or stuffy nose. _____

f. A contagious disease characterized by coughing, night sweats, decreased energy, and decreased appetite. This disease is caused by a bacterium that is inhaled and usually affects the lungs by destroying parts of the lung tissue, which is then replaced by fibrous connective tissue. _____

Vocabulary test

Match each word to its correct definition, and write your answers in the spaces provided.

WORD	DEFINITION
1. Nares	**a.** Pharyngeal tonsils
2. Cough	**b.** Also called the Adam's Apple
3. Stridor	**c.** Coughing up of blood
4. Dyspnea	**d.** A high-pitched whistling sound produced when the airways are partially obstructed
5. Hypoxia	**e.** A sudden, explosive movement of air rushing upward through the respiratory passages
6. Hemoptysis	**f.** Material coughed up from the respiratory tract
7. Sinus	**g.** Nostrils
8. Cilia	**h.** Labored or difficult breathing
9. Adenoids	**i.** Hairlike projections that line the respiratory passages and move dust-laden mucus toward the pharynx
10. Epiglottis	**j.** The inefficient delivery of oxygen to the tissues
11. Thyroid cartilage	**k.** Air-filled spaces within the facial and cranial bones
12. Sputum	**l.** A ring-shaped piece of cartilage that protects the opening of the larynx

Answers:

1. _____   2. _____   3. _____   4. _____   5. _____   6. _____   7. _____   8. _____

9. _____   10. _____   11. _____   12. _____

Multiple-Choice Questions

1. Which body system does the respiratory system work closely with to ensure there is a continuous supply of oxygen to all cells and a continuous removal of carbon dioxide?
   a. Cardiovascular system
   b. Endocrine system
   c. Lymphatic system
   d. Urinary system

2. What is the correct term used to describe the exchange of gases?
   a. Desquamation
   b. Oxidation
   c. Respiration
   d. Ventilation

3. When does blood gain oxygen and lose carbon dioxide?
   a. During pulmonary ventilation
   b. During external respiration
   c. During internal respiration
   d. During oxidation

4. When does blood lose oxygen and gain carbon dioxide?
   a. During pulmonary ventilation
   b. During external respiration
   c. During internal respiration
   d. During oxidation

5. Which of the following structures are all resonating chambers for sound?
   a. Nasal cavity, paranasal sinuses, and bronchi
   b. Mouth, trachea, lungs, bronchi, and larynx
   c. Nasal vestibule, nasal cavity, alveoli, and paranasal sinuses
   d. Pharynx, mouth, nasal cavity, and paranasal sinuses

6. What is another term for nostrils?
   a. External nares
   b. Internal nares
   c. Nasal vestibules
   d. Nasal conchae

7. Which of the following are all regions of the pharynx?
   a. Conchae, nasopharynx, larynx
   b. Oropharynx, sinuses, hypopharynx
   c. Nasopharynx, oropharynx, laryngopharynx
   d. Oropharynx, larynx, laryngopharynx

8. Which of the following best describes the structure of the larynx?
   a. A funnel-shaped tube whose walls are made up of skeletal muscles lined by mucous membrane and cilia
   b. A short passageway made up of eight pieces of rigid hyaline cartilage and a leaf-shaped piece of elastic cartilage
   c. A long, tubular passageway composed of 16–20 incomplete C-shaped rings of hyaline cartilage
   d. A short passageway composed of repeatedly dividing branches of incomplete rings of cartilage lined with a mucous membrane

9. Which of the following is incorrect?
   a. The choanae are commonly called the nostrils
   b. The pharynx is commonly called the throat
   c. The larynx is commonly called the voice box
   d. The trachea is commonly called the windpipe

10. **What is the main function of the trachea?**
    a. Routes air and food into their correct channels
    b. Produces sound
    c. Acts as a passageway for air, food, and drink
    d. Transports air

11. **Which of the following correctly depicts the branching of the bronchi?**
    a. Secondary bronchi, tertiary bronchi, bronchioles, primary bronchi
    b. Tertiary bronchi, secondary bronchi, primary bronchi, bronchioles
    c. Bronchioles, primary bronchi, tertiary bronchi, secondary bronchi
    d. Primary bronchi, secondary bronchi, tertiary bronchi, bronchioles

12. **What is the name of the membrane that covers the lungs?**
    a. Parietal pleura
    b. Visceral pleura
    c. Parietal peritoneum
    d. Visceral peritoneum

13. **Where does the gaseous exchange between the lungs and the blood occur?**
    a. At the pleura
    b. At the mediastinum
    c. At the respiratory membrane
    d. At the bronchi

14. **When does inspiration occur?**
    a. When the pressure within the lungs is lower than the pressure outside the lungs
    b. When the pressure within the lungs is higher than the pressure outside the lungs
    c. When the pressure within the lungs is equal to the pressure outside the lungs
    d. When there is no pressure within the lungs

15. **In external respiration, how does the exchange of gases take place?**
    a. Via simple diffusion
    b. Via osmosis
    c. Via facilitated diffusion
    d. Via vesicular transport

9 The Cardiovascular System

Review/Self–Study Notes

....

Blood

1. Blood is a vital substance in the body that functions in transportation, regulation, and protection. Describe each of these functions in more detail.

   • Transportation _____

   _____

   _____

   • Regulation _____

   _____

   _____

   • Protection _____

   _____

   _____

2. The heart has four valves, which prevent blood from flowing backward. In the spaces provided below create your own mnemonic to remind you of each valve and its function.
   • **Atrioventricular (AV) valves** lie between the atria and the ventricles and prevent blood from flowing back into the atria when the ventricles contract.
     ○ **Tricuspid valve**—right AV valve

   Mnemonic: _____

     ○ **Mitral valve**—left AV valve

   Mnemonic: _____

- **Semilunar valves** lie between the ventricles and the arteries and prevent blood from flowing back into the ventricles when they relax.
  - ○ **Pulmonary semilunar valve**—between the right ventricle and the pulmonary trunk

Mnemonic: _____

  - ○ **Aortic semilunar valve**—between the left ventricle and the aorta

Mnemonic: _____

The heart

3. Color and label the following diagram of the heart.

KEY: THE HEART		
Structure	**Description/Function**	**Color**
Inferior vena cava		
Superior vena cava		
Right atrium		
Right ventricle		
Pulmonary artery		
Pulmonary veins		
Left atrium		
Left ventricle		
Aorta		
Descending aorta		

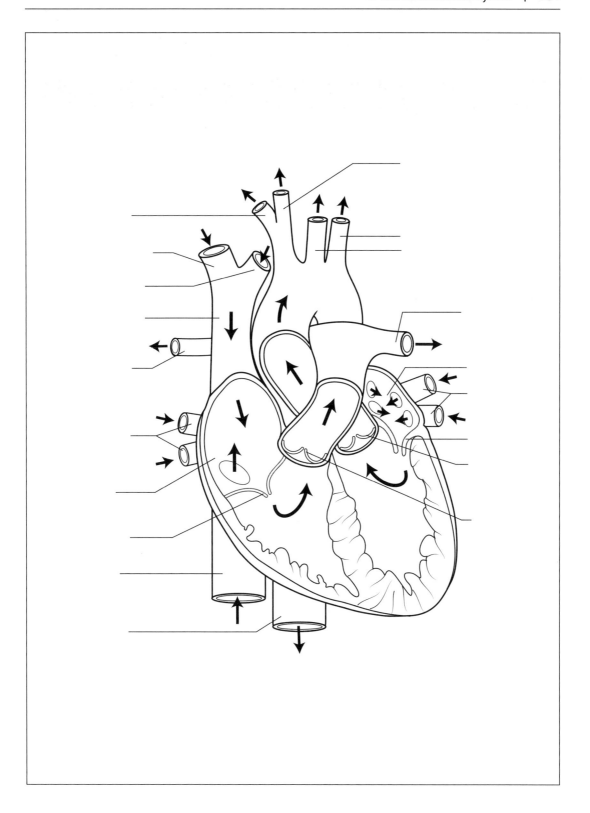

4. The heart is a "double pump" because it pumps blood into two different circulations: pulmonary circulation and systemic circulation. Color and label the diagram below.

KEY: PULMONARY AND SYSTEMIC CIRCULATION		
Structure	**Description/Function**	**Color**
Veins		
Right atrium		
Right ventricle		
Pulmonary arteries		
Pulmonary capillaries		
Pulmonary veins		
Left atrium		
Left ventricle		
Arteries		
Systemic capillaries		

Physiology of the heart

5. To ensure that you really understand what makes the heart beat and what controls or affects the heartbeat, put yourself in the examiner's seat and write questions on the topics given below. Then put yourself back in your own seat and answer the questions.

Study tip
....

You may find it easier and more interesting if you do this exercise as part of a group.

---

a. Ask a question on the intrinsic conduction system (nodal system).

Question: _____

Answer: _____

_____

_____

b. Ask a question on the regulation of the heart rate.

Question: _____

Answer: _____

_____

_____

c. Ask a question on the cardiac cycle.

Question: _____

Answer: _____

_____

_____

d. Ask a question about blood pressure.

Question: _____

Answer: _____

_____

_____

Blood vessels

6. The cardiovascular system is composed of a closed system of tubes that all connect with one another to transport blood around the body. Complete the table below on the different types of blood vessels.

Vessel	Structure	Transports Blood From	Transports Blood To
Artery			
Arteriole			
Capillary			
Vein			
Venule			

7. The heart is a double pump that pumps blood into two different circulations: pulmonary circulation and systemic circulation. In addition to this, there are two other recognized circulations: coronary circulation and hepatic portal circulation. In the spaces provided, draw a spider diagram or mind map of each of these circulations.

8. Now it's time to use your imagination! In order to learn the names of the many blood vessels in the body, picture it as a map and think of all the vessels as roads. A friend of yours is lost and needs directions, so, giving each vessel a road name, direct your friend around the body.

Study tip

You may find it easier and more interesting if you do this exercise as part of a group. Have fun: create highways, roads, avenues, lanes and maybe even footpaths for the capillaries. You can either write the directions or draw them if you prefer.

Common pathologies of the cardiovascular system

9. Write down a short phrase that will remind you of each of the following diseases and disorders.

Blood disorders:

- Iron-deficiency anemia _____

- Pernicious anemia _____

- Sickle-cell anemia _____

- Dyslipidemia _____

- Epistaxis (nosebleeds) _____

- Hematoma _____

- Hemophilia _____

- Thrombophilia _____

- Thrombosis _____

- Coronary thrombosis _____

- Deep vein thrombosis _____

- Pulmonary embolism _____

- Septicemia _____

- Thalassemia _____

Heart and blood-vessel disorders:

- Aneurysm _____

- Angina pectoris _____

- Arrhythmia _____

- Arteriosclerosis _____

- Atherosclerosis _____

- Cardiac failure _____

- Coronary artery disease _____

- Gangrene _____

- Hemorrhoids (piles) _____

- Hypertension _____

- Hypotension _____

- Intermittent claudication _____

- Myocardial infarction (heart attack)

  _____

- Palpitations and panic attacks _____

- Phlebitis _____

- Raynaud's disease _____

- Septal defect (hole in the heart) _____

- Varicose veins (varices) _____

Exercises

1. Complete the crossword below.

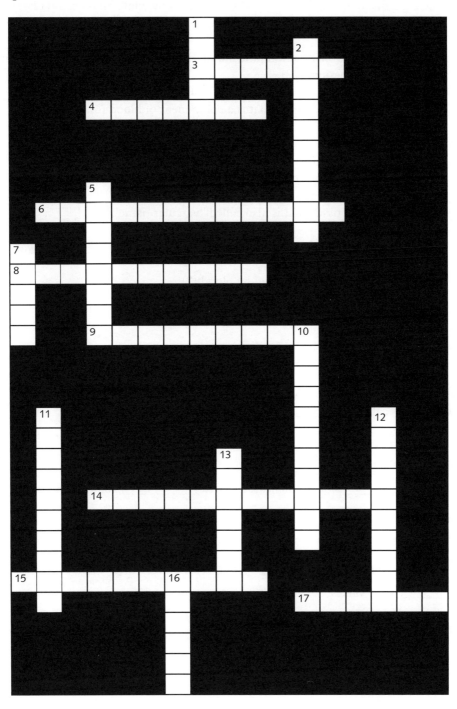

Across:

3. Organ that filters, cleans, and stores blood (6).
4. The function that water performs in blood (7).
6. The engulfment and digestion of foreign particles by white blood cells (12).
8. A white blood cell that plays an important role in the immune response (10).
9. A white blood cell (9).
14. Charged particles (ions) found in the blood. Examples include sodium, potassium, calcium, and magnesium (12).
15. A protein that functions in blood clotting (10).
17. A watery, straw-colored liquid that is a component of blood (6).

Down:

1. What blood removes from cells (5).
2. The oxygen-carrying molecule in blood (10).
5. A granulocyte that releases histamine (8).
7. A fluid connective tissue that is also called "vascular tissue" (5).
10. A red blood cell (11).
11. A white blood cell that engulfs and digests foreign particles and removes waste (10).
12. The stopping of bleeding (10).
13. A chemical messenger transported by blood (7).
16. Gas that is carried by red blood cells (6).

2. **Fill in the missing words.**

   a. The heart is a hollow, muscular organ divided into two halves. Both halves receive and deliver blood. The receiving chamber is called an _____ and the delivering chamber is called a _____.

   b. The _____ side of the heart receives _____ blood from the body and pumps it to the _____.

   c. The _____ side of the heart receives _____ blood from the lungs and pumps it to the _____.

   d. Separating the chambers of the heart are valves. Their main function is to prevent blood from flowing _____. These valves are the _____ valves and the _____ valves.

3. The table below summarizes the principal blood vessels of the heart. Complete the table.

Vessel	Blood	From	To
Aorta	a.	b.	Most of the body
Coronary artery	Oxygenated	c.	d.
Pulmonary artery	e.	Heart	f.
Superior vena cava	Deoxygenated	g.	h.
Inferior vena cava	i.	j.	Heart
Coronary sinus	k.	Heart tissue	Heart
Pulmonary vein	l.	m.	Heart

4. Use the clues below to unscramble the following letters.

a. ESORNITAALINDO _____

b. YOSSETL _____

c. YDRCAAICCCLE _____

d. SATUHORTILHCMCLEY _____

e. LOERATREIS _____

f. LESIDAOT _____

Clues (note, these are not in order):
- Specialized cells that form the pacemaker of the heart
- A mass of autorhythmic cells found in the right atrial wall that initiate impulses and so start each heartbeat
- All the events associated with a heartbeat
- Contraction
- Relaxation
- Small vessels that carry blood away from the heart toward the tissues

5. **Dave is a young adult male whose blood pressure is 160/100 mm Hg.**

    a. Is Dave's blood pressure considered normal? If not, what is considered to be a normal

    blood pressure? _____

    _____

    b. Explain to Dave what the first figure, 160, and the second figure, 100, represent.

    _____

    _____

6. **Match the names of the blood vessels below to their descriptions, and write the answers in the spaces provided.**

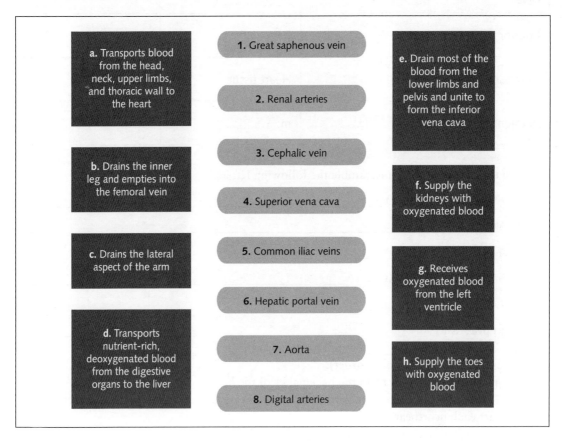

a. Transports blood from the head, neck, upper limbs, and thoracic wall to the heart

b. Drains the inner leg and empties into the femoral vein

c. Drains the lateral aspect of the arm

d. Transports nutrient-rich, deoxygenated blood from the digestive organs to the liver

1. Great saphenous vein

2. Renal arteries

3. Cephalic vein

4. Superior vena cava

5. Common iliac veins

6. Hepatic portal vein

7. Aorta

8. Digital arteries

e. Drain most of the blood from the lower limbs and pelvis and unite to form the inferior vena cava

f. Supply the kidneys with oxygenated blood

g. Receives oxygenated blood from the left ventricle

h. Supply the toes with oxygenated blood

Answers:

1. _____ 2. _____ 3. _____ 4. _____ 5. _____ 6. _____ 7. _____ 8. _____

Common pathologies of the cardiovascular system

7. Are the following statements true or false? Write T or F in the spaces provided.

   a. Anemia is an increase in the oxygen-carrying capacity of the blood. _____

   b. Hemophilia is a hereditary disorder in which blood clots very slowly. _____

   c. Deep vein thrombosis is the blocking of the pulmonary artery by an embolus. _____

   d. The clinical term for nosebleeds is arrhythmia. _____

   e. The clinical term for a heart attack is myocardial infarction. _____

   f. Edema is the excessive accumulation of interstitial fluid in body tissues. _____

   g. Arteriosclerosis is the death and decay of tissue due to a lack of blood supply. _____

   h. The common name for hypotension is high blood pressure. _____

   i. Phlebitis is the inflammation of the walls of a vein. _____

   j. Raynaud's disease is the temporary sensation of a chest pain caused by a lack of oxygen to the heart muscle. _____

Red flags

8. If a person presents with the following signs and symptoms, what condition should you suspect?

   a. Rapid breathing with fever, chills, shaking, and a warm skin. Patient also appears somewhat confused. **Answer:** _____

   b. Numbness or weakness on one side of the body, with slurred speech, mental confusion, and loss of balance. **Answer:** _____

   c. Rapid breathing with weakness, fatigue, dizziness, and a cool, clammy skin. Patient also appears very anxious. **Answer:** _____

   d. Chest pain accompanied by shortness of breath, sweating, and anxiety.

   Answer: _____

Vocabulary test

9. Give the correct medical term of the following more commonly used names:

   a. Heart attack _____

   b. Slow heart rate _____

   c. Piles _____

   d. Bleeding from nose _____

   e. Blood clot _____

   f. High blood pressure _____

10. Complete the table below.

WORD	DEFINITION
Diastole	a. _____
Systole	b. _____
Vasoconstriction	c. _____
Vasodilation	d. _____

Multiple-Choice Questions

1. What type of tissue is blood?
   a. Epithelial
   b. Connective
   c. Muscle
   d. Nervous

2. Which of the following are all functions of blood?
   a. Transportation, regulation, protection
   b. Protection, locomotion, metabolism
   c. Metabolism, excretion, thermogenesis
   d. Excretion, locomotion, regulation

3. Which of the following are all types of white blood cells?
   a. Erythrocytes, neutrophils, lymphocytes
   b. Thrombocytes, plasma, hemoglobin
   c. Basophils, eosinophils, monocytes
   d. Fibrinogen, globulins, albumins

4. What is the name of the chamber of the heart that receives blood?
   a. Atrium
   b. Ventricle
   c. Pericardium
   d. Apex

5. What is the name of the triple-layered sac that surrounds and protects the heart?
   a. Pleura
   b. Perineum
   c. Peritoneum
   d. Pericardium

6. How many compartments, or chambers, is the heart divided into?
   a. 1
   b. 2
   c. 3
   d. 4

7. Which valves lie between the atria and ventricles and prevent blood from flowing back into the atria when the ventricles contract?
   a. Atrioventricular valves
   b. Semilunar valves
   c. Interventricular valves
   d. Bilunar valves

8. Which side of the heart receives deoxygenated blood from the body and pumps it to the lungs?
   a. Right
   b. Left
   c. Both
   d. None of the above

9. What is the name of the vessels that carry blood away from the tissues toward the heart?
   a. Arteries
   b. Arterioles
   c. Capillaries
   d. Veins

10. Which type of blood vessel has walls that are composed of a single layer of endothelium and a basement membrane?
    a. Arteries
    b. Arterioles
    c. Capillaries
    d. Veins

11. Which of the following statements is true?
    a. The structure of veins is the same as that of arteries
    b. The walls of veins are thinner than those of arteries and some veins have valves to prevent the backflow of blood as it flows up toward the heart

c. The lumens of arteries are smaller than those of veins and some arteries have valves to prevent the backflow of blood as it flows away from the heart

d. Veins consist of a triple-layered wall surrounding a lumen, while arteries consist of a double-layered wall surrounding a lumen

12. Which of the following statements best describes the flow of blood through vessels?
   a. Blood flows from an area of high pressure into an area of low pressure
   b. Blood flows from an area of low pressure into an area of high pressure
   c. Blood flows from an area of high pressure into an area of equal pressure
   d. Blood flows from an area of low pressure into an area of equal pressure

13. What is the name of the route blood follows from the heart to the tissues and organs of the body and back to the heart?
   a. Coronary circulation
   b. Pulmonary circulation
   c. Renal circulation
   d. Systemic circulation

14. Which of the following blood vessels descend into the thighs to become the femoral arteries?
   a. Popliteal arteries
   b. Popliteal veins
   c. Internal iliac arteries
   d. External iliac arteries

15. Which of the following blood vessels receives blood from the head, neck, upper limbs, and thoracic wall?
   a. Superior phrenic artery
   b. Inferior phrenic vein
   c. Superior vena cava
   d. Inferior vena cava

10 The Lymphatic and Immune System

Review/Self–Study Notes

The lymphatic system

1. The lymphatic system has three main functions. It drains interstitial fluid, transports dietary lipids, and protects against invasions. Describe each of these functions in your own words.

- Drains interstitial fluid _____

_____

_____

_____

_____

_____

- Transports dietary lipids _____

_____

_____

_____

_____

_____

- Protects against invasions _____

_____

_____

_____

_____

_____

2. The lymphatic system is composed of a number of different vessels and structures through which lymph passes on its way to the subclavian veins. This journey has been outlined for you below. Create a spider diagram or mind map of the journey of lymph from interstitial fluid to its final destination.

   Interstitial fluid → lymphatic capillaries → lymphatic vessels → lymphatic trunks → lymphatic ducts → subclavian veins

   Once you have traced this journey, add in the following structures, and next to each structure describe its function.
   • Lymph nodes
   • Thymus gland
   • Spleen
   • Lymphatic nodules

3. Color and label the following diagrams related to the lymphatic system.

KEY: A LYMPH NODE		
Structure	**Function/Description**	**Color**
Afferent lymphatic vessels		
Efferent lymphatic vessels		
One-way valves		
Capsule		
Trabeculae		
Reticular tissue		
Follicles		
Cortex		
Medulla		

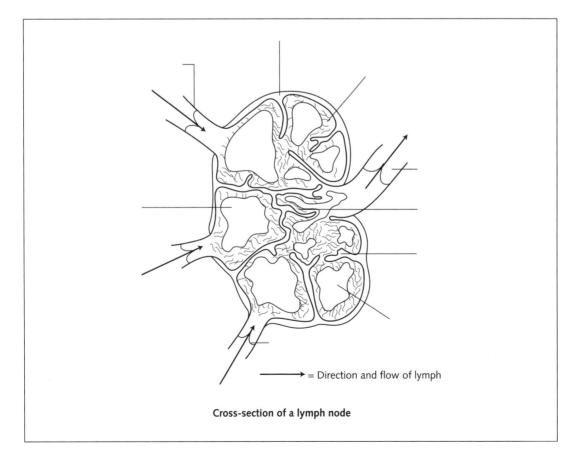

→ = Direction and flow of lymph

Cross-section of a lymph node

KEY: THE LYMPHATIC SYSTEM		
Structure	Function/Description	Color
Lymphatic organs and nodules (mucosa-associated lymphoid tissue)		
Tonsils		
Thymus		
Spleen		
Aggregated lymphatic follicles (Peyer's patches) Note: Although only a few are shown here, there are many distributed throughout the ileum		
Appendix		
Bone marrow		
Lymph nodes		
Lymph nodes of the head (includes the parotid, auricular, mastoid, submandibular, submental, and occipital nodes)		
Cervical lymph nodes		
Axillary lymph nodes		
Supratrochlear nodes		
Iliac nodes		
Inguinal nodes		
Popliteal nodes Note: These nodes are behind the knee, not in front of it		
Other important lymphatic structures		
Thoracic duct		
Cisterna chyle		

Internal jugular vein

Subclavian vein

Femur

KEY: LYMPHATIC ORGANS		
Structure	Function/Description	Color
Tonsils and adenoids		
Thymus		
Mucosa-associated lymphoid tissue (MALT) of lungs		
Spleen		
Peyer's patches		
Appendix		
Bone marrow		

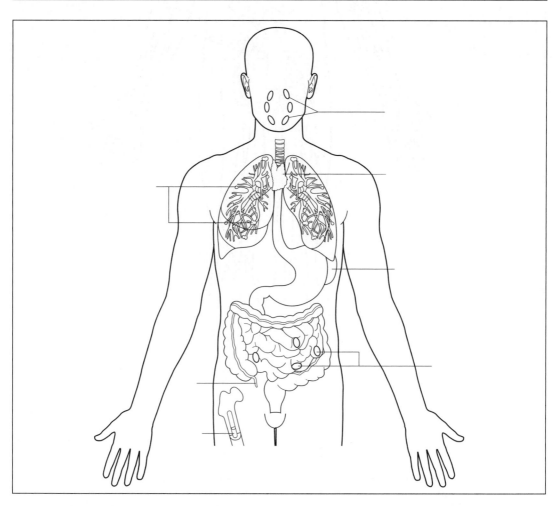

Resistance to disease and immunity

Our body is constantly being attacked by a multitude of invaders and it defends itself in two different ways—through non-specific resistance to disease and through the immune response (immunity).

4. Imagine you are the general of an army that will attack a healthy person's body. You have different army personnel you can use, but you firstly need to inform them of what lies ahead. They know nothing about the body they are going to attack and you need to teach them about the different lines of defense they will encounter. Following is a list of what you need to include. In the box beneath, either write notes or sketch images that give details of each line of defense.

First Line of Defense	Specialized Defense
Mechanical barriers Chemical barriers Natural killer cells Phagocytes Inflammation Fever	Immunocompetent cells Immune responses Immunological memory

Study tip
....

You may find it easier and more interesting if you do this exercise as part of a group. You can make more of this exercise by taking time to discuss what could weaken a healthy body's defenses; for example, poor nutrition, lack of exercise, stress.

Common pathologies of the lymphatic and immune system

Red flags

5. Describe the signs and symptoms of anaphylaxis. _____

   _____

   _____

   _____

   _____

6. Write down a short phrase that will remind you of each of the following pathologies of the lymphatic and immune system.

   • Allergy _____

   _____

   _____

   • Lymphadenitis _____

   _____

   _____

   • Lymphedema _____

   _____

   _____

   Cancer and the lymphatic and immune system:

   • Leukemia _____

   _____

   _____

• Lymphoma _____

   _____

   _____

• Hodgkin's disease _____

   _____

   _____

• Non-Hodgkin's lymphoma _____

   _____

   _____

Infectious diseases:

• Acquired immunodeficiency syndrome (AIDS) _____

   _____

   _____

• Glandular fever (infectious mononucleosis) _____

   _____

   _____

• Tonsillitis _____

   _____

   _____

Autoimmune diseases and disorders:

• Systemic lupus erythematosus (SLE)

   _____

   _____

Exercises

1. **List the three main functions of the lymphatic system.**

   • _____

   • _____

   • _____

2. **Are the following statements true or false? Write T or F in the spaces provided.**

   a. Lymph is a clear fluid derived from interstitial fluid. It contains protein molecules, lipid molecules, and red blood cells. _____

   b. Lymph is only found in lymphatic vessels. _____

   c. Interstitial fluid is absorbed into lymphatic capillaries where it becomes lymph. These capillaries transport it into lymphatic vessels, which carry it through a number of lymph nodes and then into larger vessels called lymphatic trunks. _____

   d. Lymphatic trunks carry lymph into two main ducts. The thoracic duct receives lymph from the upper right side of the body and the right lymphatic duct receives lymph from the entire body below the ribs. _____

   e. Lymph nodes can also be called lymph glands. _____

3. **Match the lymphatic structures to their functions and write the answers in the spaces provided below.**

a. Lymph nodes	**1.** Filters and stores blood, destroys old worn-out red blood cells, and produces lymphocytes
b. Thymus gland	**2.** Help protect the body from pathogens that have been inhaled, digested, or have entered the body via external openings
c. Spleen	**3.** Produces hormones that help the development and maturation of T cells
d. Lymphatic nodules	**4.** Filter lymph and produce lymphocytes

Answers:

1. _____   2. _____   3. _____   4. _____

4. **The word search contains the names of different lymph nodes. Use the locations given below to find these names.**

K	D	S	U	P	R	A	T	R	O	C	H	L	E	A	R	A	S	H
G	J	R	O	F	D	B	D	R	I	Y	A	D	X	N	I	R	P	O
S	U	P	E	R	F	I	C	I	A	L	P	A	R	O	T	I	D	N
U	S	G	E	D	A	P	Z	G	X	N	J	K	T	C	K	G	V	Y
B	Y	Y	Q	E	T	I	L	L	I	L	G	D	S	C	E	F	G	F
M	D	M	A	S	T	O	I	D	L	F	Q	Y	E	I	Q	W	H	S
A	K	L	D	U	A	S	F	G	L	G	A	F	W	P	Y	T	H	M
N	V	W	H	B	F	D	G	E	A	Y	E	U	Q	I	I	H	E	C
D	L	Z	E	M	H	J	J	D	R	G	D	K	D	T	J	X	W	P
I	W	W	X	E	C	K	J	O	Y	F	Y	J	A	A	G	W	N	O
B	R	R	X	N	K	L	G	U	Y	D	H	K	D	L	T	E	M	P
U	F	H	H	T	U	I	L	E	O	C	O	L	I	C	S	J	S	L
L	M	O	U	A	Y	L	R	H	Y	D	G	F	D	B	C	A	O	I
A	G	D	I	L	G	I	C	E	R	V	I	C	A	L	B	S	I	T
R	O	Y	O	A	D	A	A	M	D	H	R	S	G	E	R	R	C	E
C	I	E	K	W	L	C	S	G	C	R	F	D	Y	Y	Y	J	S	A
D	U	G	M	S	N	T	D	H	I	N	G	U	I	N	A	L	V	L

Location of lymph node:
- In front of ears
- Behind ears
- Beneath mandible
- Beneath chin
- Base of skull
- Neck
- Armpit
- Elbow crease
- Abdomen (near the diaphragm)
- Abdomen
- Groin
- Behind the knee

5. The body employs two different approaches to defend itself against invaders. The first approach is non-specific resistance to disease. The second is the immune response. Each of these approaches uses a variety of different mechanisms, all given below. Link these mechanisms to their approaches.

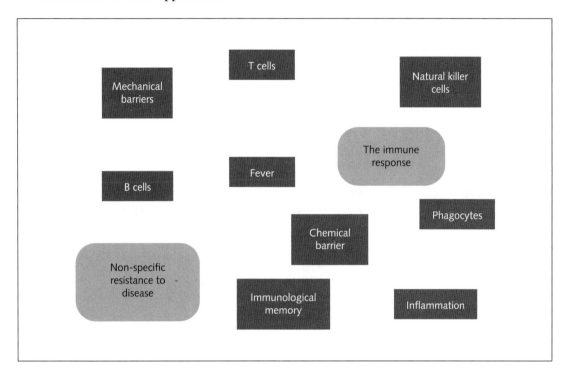

Common pathologies of the lymphatic and immune system

6. Name the following diseases and disorders.

   a. Excessive swelling due to an accumulation of lymph in the tissues _____

   b. Cancer of the white blood cells _____

   c. A malignant lymphoma characterized by the progressive, painless enlargement of lymph nodes _____

   d. A disease caused by the human immunodeficiency virus that results in a lowered T4 lymphocyte count and greater susceptibility to infections

   _____

   e. Also called infectious mononucleosis, this disease is characterized by fatigue, headaches, dizziness, and enlarged and tender lymph nodes

   _____

7. **Match the correct word to its definition, and write the answers in the spaces provided.**

1. Lysozyme	**a.** Specialized lymphatic vessel located in the villi of the small intestine; it absorbs lipids and lipid-soluble vitamins
2. Interferon	**b.** A collection of proteins that act sequentially to enhance the body's primary defense mechanisms
3. Natural killer cell	**c.** Type of white blood cell involved in immunity; for example, B cells and T cells
4. Lacteal	**d.** Fluid found in the spaces around cells
5. Complement system	**e.** Type of lymphocyte that can kill a variety of microbes as well as some tumor cells
6. Lymphocyte	**f.** Enzyme found in certain body secretions such as tears and saliva; it catalyzes the breakdown of the cell walls of certain bacteria
7. Interstitial fluid	**g.** Substance produced to protect uninfected cells from viral infection

Answers:

1. _____ 2. _____ 3. _____ 4. _____ 5. _____ 6. _____ 7. _____

Vocabulary test

Complete the table below.

WORD	DEFINITION	
Antibody	**a.**	_____
Antigen	**b.**	_____
Macrophage	**c.**	_____
Metastasis	**d.**	_____
Phagocyte	**e.**	_____

Multiple-Choice Questions

1. Which of the following best describes an antigen?
   a. A specialized protein that is synthesized to destroy foreign particles
   b. A substance that the body recognizes as foreign
   c. A scavenger cell that engulfs and destroys foreign particles
   d. A disease-causing microorganism

2. Which of the following is not a function of the lymphatic system?
   a. Immune response
   b. Drainage of interstitial fluid
   c. Thermogenesis
   d. Transportation of fats

3. Which of the following are transported by the lymphatic system?
   a. Vitamins A, D, E, and K
   b. Calcium, magnesium, and zinc
   c. Carbohydrates
   d. Red blood cells

4. Where in the body do some lymphocytes become immune competent?
   a. Liver
   b. Thymus
   c. Brain
   d. Kidneys

5. What is another name for lymphatic nodules?
   a. Lymphatic vessels
   b. Lymph nodes
   c. Lymphatic trunks
   d. Mucosa-associated lymphoid tissue

6. Which of the following are all found in lymph?
   a. Protein molecules, lipid molecules, foreign particles, cell debris, lymphocytes
   b. Lipid molecules, bacteria, dead cells, erythrocytes
   c. Platelets, bacteria, erythrocytes, dead cells
   d. Foreign particles, cell debris, lymphocytes, erythrocytes

7. Where do the lymphatic ducts empty their contents?
   a. Into lymphatic trunks
   b. Into the left and right subclavian veins
   c. Into lymphatic capillaries
   d. Into the left and right carotid veins

8. Which of the following do not help lymph move through the lymphatic vessels?
   a. Breathing movements
   b. Skeletal muscle
   c. B and T cells
   d. One-way valves

9. What is the function of lymph nodes?
   a. To filter and clean blood
   b. To protect the external openings of the body
   c. To store platelets and blood
   d. To filter lymph and produce lymphocytes

10. What structure can be described as follows: located on the left side of the body, this structure consists of white pulp and red pulp enclosed in a dense connective tissue from which trabeculae extend to form its framework?
    a. Lymph nodes
    b. Lymphatic nodules
    c. Thymus
    d. Spleen

11. Where in the body are lymphatic nodules found?
    a. Gastrointestinal tract and respiratory airways
    b. Liver and large intestine
    c. Heart and brain
    d. Reproductive tract and gall bladder

12. What are the signs and symptoms of inflammation?
    a. Swelling and heat
    b. Redness and pain
    c. Occasionally the loss of function
    d. All of the above

13. Which of the following are all mechanical barriers to disease?
    a. Sebum and saliva
    b. Lacrimal apparatus and gastric juice
    c. The skin and urination
    d. Perspiration and vaginal secretions

14. What type of cell are macrophages?
    a. Erythrocytes
    b. Platelets
    c. Natural killer cells
    d. Phagocytes

15. What happens during an antibody-mediated immune response?
    a. Killer cells attack antigens
    b. Antibodies attack antigens
    c. Phagocytes attack antigens
    d. Macrophages attack antigens

11 The Digestive System

Review/Self–Study Notes

1. Describe the basic processes and functions of the digestive system.

   • Ingestion _____

   • Secretion _____

   • Mixing and propulsion _____

   • Mechanical digestion _____

   • Chemical digestion _____

   • Absorption _____

   • Defecation _____

2. Describe the structure of the wall of the gastrointestinal tract.

   _____

   _____

3. The digestive system may seem daunting. However, it is actually quite straightforward. You just need to learn the different structures of the system and what they do. Make some flash cards. On the front of the card write the name of the structure or organ and on the back write its function. Here is an example of a flash card for the mouth:

Mouth	**Mechanical digestion:** Mastication Deglutition **Chemical digestion:** Salivary amylase (carbohydrates) Lingual lipase (lipids)

Ensure you include these organs and structures of the gastrointestinal tract:
• Mouth
• Pharynx
• Esophagus
• Stomach
• Small intestine (duodenum, jejunum, and ileum)
• Large intestine
• Anus

And these accessory structures:
• Teeth, tongue, salivary glands
• Liver
• Gall bladder
• Pancreas

Study groups

....

To help you revise the digestive system use your flash cards to play the game "30 seconds." Turn to chapter 1 to learn how to play.

4. Color and label the diagrams below of the digestive system.

KEY: THE DIGESTIVE SYSTEM		
Structure	Function	Color
Mouth		
Salivary glands (parotid, submandibular, and sublingual)		
Epiglottis		
Esophagus		
Stomach		
Pancreas		
Liver		
Gall bladder		
Small intestine (duodenum, jejunum, ileum)		
Large intestine (cecum, ascending colon, transverse colon, descending colon, sigmoid colon, rectum, anal canal)		

KEY: THE TEETH		
Structure	**Function**	**Color**
Incisors		
Canines		
Premolars		
Molars		

Permanent (secondary) dentition

Deciduous (primary) dentition

5. Now that you know the basic structure and function of the digestive system, you need to learn about the digestion of carbohydrates, proteins, and lipids. In the spaces below, draw a spider diagram or mind map to show the digestion of each of these.

Study tip
....

Be imaginative and have fun—the more you enjoy what you are doing the easier you will remember it. Use color, symbols, images, and even rhymes.

Digestion of carbohydrates

Digestion of proteins

Digestion of lipids

Common pathologies of the digestive system

6. **Write down a short phrase that will remind you of each of the following diseases or disorders.**

   Pathologies of the mouth and teeth:

   - Apical abscess (tooth abscess) _____

   - Gingivitis _____

   - Halitosis _____

   Pathologies of the esophagus and stomach:

   - Dyspepsia (indigestion) _____

   - Heartburn _____

   - Hiatus hernia _____

   - Hiccups _____

   - Gastric ulcer _____

   - Gastro-esophageal reflux disease (GERD) _____

   - Esophagitis _____

   Pathologies of the liver, gall bladder, and pancreas:

   - Cholecystitis _____

   - Cirrhosis of the liver _____

   - Gallstones _____

   - Hepatitis _____

   - Hepatitis A _____

   - Hepatitis B _____

   - Hepatitis C _____

   - Pancreatitis _____

Pathologies of the small and large intestines:

- Appendicitis _____

- Celiac disease _____

- Colitis _____

- Colon cancer (colorectal cancer)

  _____

- Constipation _____

- Diarrhea _____

- Diverticulosis _____

- Diverticulitis _____

- Enteritis _____

- Flatulence _____

- Gastritis _____

- Gastroenteritis _____

- Inflammatory bowel disease (IBD)

  _____

- Crohn's disease _____

- Ulcerative colitis _____

- Irritable bowel syndrome (IBS)

  _____

- Peptic ulcer _____

Eating disorders:

- Anorexia nervosa _____

- Bulimia nervosa _____

- Obesity _____

Exercises

1. Complete the crossword.

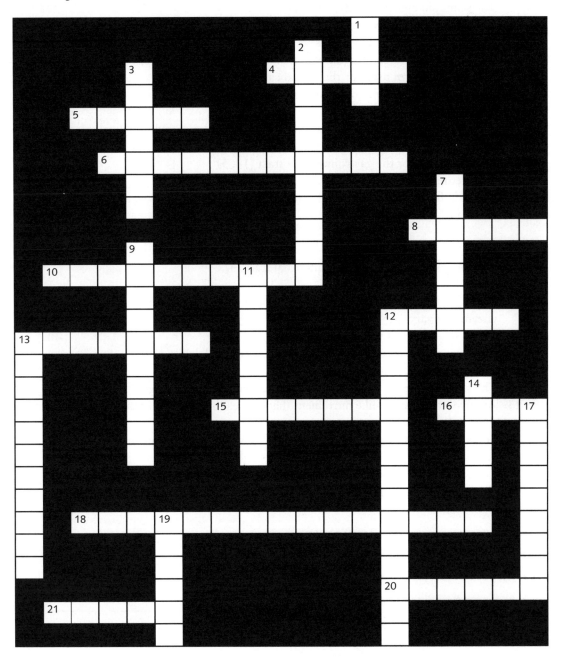

Across:

4. The pouch at the start of the large intestine that receives food from the small intestine (6).
5. The semifluid contents of the stomach (5).
6. Another term for chewing (11).
8. Another name for the large intestine (5).
10. The process by which indigestible substances are eliminated from the body (10).
12. The common term used for the buccal cavity (5).
13. Salivary glands below and in front of the ear (7).
15. The enzymes that digest fats (7).
16. A brownish yellow liquid that is produced by the liver, stored in the gall bladder, and necessary for the digestion of fats (4).
18. Another name for the gastrointestinal tract (10, 5)
20. Another term used for teeth (6).
21. The soft, flexible mass that food is reduced to after being chewed and mixed with saliva (5).

Down:

1. Terminal opening of the gastrointestinal tract (4).
2. The act of swallowing (11).
3. The digestion of starches begins in the mouth when they come into contact with the enzyme salivary _____ (7).
7. The first segment of the small intestine (8).
9. The large serous membrane that lines the abdominal cavity (10).
11. The process of taking food into the mouth (9).
12. The molecules carbohydrates are broken down into during digestion (15).
13. An involuntary wave-like movement that pushes the contents of the gastrointestinal tract forward (11).
14. Functions of this vital organ include metabolism, detoxification, and nutrient storage (5).
17. Long tube running behind the trachea (10).
19. The name of the deepest layer of the wall of the gastrointestinal tract (6).

2. The columns below show the major digestive organs and the enzymes/fluids that are found within them. However, some of these enzymes are in the wrong columns. Cross out those that are in the incorrect columns and write their names in the correct columns.

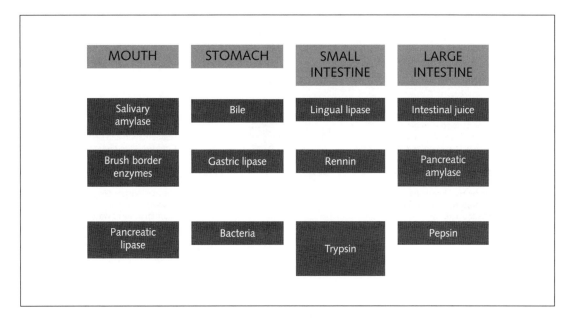

3. Are the following statements true or false? Write T or F in the spaces provided.

   a. The digestion of carbohydrates begins in the mouth and is completed in the small intestine. _____

   b. The digestion of proteins begins in the mouth and is completed in the stomach. _____

   c. Maltase, sucrase, and lactase are all enzymes that digest proteins. _____

   d. Bile emulsifies fats in the small intestine. _____

   e. Lipids are absorbed in the small intestine and transported to the liver via the hepatic portal vein. _____

4. The figure below is an overview of the organs and structures of the digestive system and their functions. However, the labels are incorrect. Relabel the diagram correctly by matching the label letter (a, b, c) to its correct line number (1, 2, 3). Write your answers in the spaces provided.

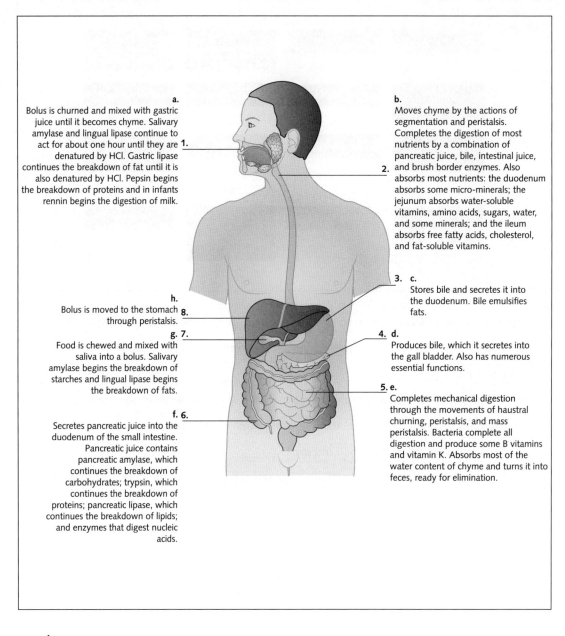

a.
Bolus is churned and mixed with gastric juice until it becomes chyme. Salivary amylase and lingual lipase continue to act for about one hour until they are denatured by HCl. Gastric lipase continues the breakdown of fat until it is also denatured by HCl. Pepsin begins the breakdown of proteins and in infants rennin begins the digestion of milk.

b.
Moves chyme by the actions of segmentation and peristalsis. Completes the digestion of most nutrients by a combination of pancreatic juice, bile, intestinal juice, and brush border enzymes. Also absorbs most nutrients: the duodenum absorbs some micro-minerals; the jejunum absorbs water-soluble vitamins, amino acids, sugars, water, and some minerals; and the ileum absorbs free fatty acids, cholesterol, and fat-soluble vitamins.

c.
Stores bile and secretes it into the duodenum. Bile emulsifies fats.

d.
Produces bile, which it secretes into the gall bladder. Also has numerous essential functions.

e.
Completes mechanical digestion through the movements of haustral churning, peristalsis, and mass peristalsis. Bacteria complete all digestion and produce some B vitamins and vitamin K. Absorbs most of the water content of chyme and turns it into feces, ready for elimination.

h.
Bolus is moved to the stomach through peristalsis.

g.
Food is chewed and mixed with saliva into a bolus. Salivary amylase begins the breakdown of starches and lingual lipase begins the breakdown of fats.

f.
Secretes pancreatic juice into the duodenum of the small intestine. Pancreatic juice contains pancreatic amylase, which continues the breakdown of carbohydrates; trypsin, which continues the breakdown of proteins; pancreatic lipase, which continues the breakdown of lipids; and enzymes that digest nucleic acids.

Answers:

1. _____   2. _____   3. _____   4. _____   5. _____   6. _____   7. _____   8. _____

Common pathologies of the digestive system

5. In the table below match the disease or disorder to its correct description and write your answers in the spaces provided.

Disease/Disorder	Description
1. Bulimia nervosa	**a.** Inflammation of the gums
2. Celiac disease	**b.** Cancer of the large intestine
3. Colorectal cancer	**c.** Psychological disorder characterized by bingeing and purging
4. Crohn's disease	**d.** Condition characterized by recurring flare-ups of abdominal pain, constipation, and diarrhea in an otherwise healthy person
5. Gingivitis	**e.** Yellowing of the skin or whites of the eyes due to high levels of bilirubin in the bloodstream
6. Hepatitis	**f.** Chronic inflammation of the wall of the gastrointestinal tract
7. Irritable bowel syndrome	**g.** Destruction of liver tissue and its replacement by scar tissue
8. Jaundice	**h.** Intolerance to gluten
9. Liver cirrhosis	**i.** A break in the mucous lining of the gastrointestinal tract usually due to the combined action of pepsin and hydrochloric acid
10. Peptic ulcer	**j.** Inflammation of the liver

Answers:

1. _____   2. _____   3. _____   4. _____   5. _____   6. _____   7. _____

8. _____   9. _____   10. _____

Red flags

6. Below are signs and symptoms that can accompany digestive disorders. Circle those that should be referred on to a medical doctor.
    a. Abdominal pain accompanied by fever, nausea, and vomiting
    b. Discomfort in the upper abdomen after eating
    c. Flatulence after a large meal
    d. Nausea accompanied by severe headache, stiff neck, and mental confusion
    e. Debilitating abdominal pain accompanied by distended abdomen, nausea, and vomiting
    f. Iron-deficiency anemia in a 54-year-old man
    g. Bad breath
    h. Bleeding of gums when brushing teeth
    i. Diarrhea accompanied by fever and blood in the stool

Vocabulary test

Complete the table below.

WORD	DEFINITION
Absorption	a.
Catalyst	b.
Digestion	c.
Substrate	d.
Jaundice	e.
Defecation	f.
Halitosis	g.
Edema	h.
Deglutition	i.
Mastication	j.

Multiple-Choice Questions

1. The functions of the digestive system can be broken down into basic processes. What is the correct order in which these processes take place?
   a. Defecation, secretion, ingestion, absorption, digestion, propulsion, mixing
   b. Ingestion, secretion, mixing, propulsion, digestion, absorption, defecation
   c. Mixing, digestion, ingestion, secretion, defecation, propulsion, absorption
   d. Absorption, ingestion, mixing, propulsion, digestion, secretion, defecation

2. Which of the following is not part of the mechanical digestion of food?
   a. Mastication
   b. Deglutition
   c. Peristalsis
   d. Enzymatic action

3. Which of the following are all part of the gastrointestinal tract?
   a. Mouth, pharynx, esophagus, stomach, intestines
   b. Mouth, teeth, tongue, esophagus, intestines
   c. Pharynx, gall bladder, liver, pancreas
   d. Gall bladder, esophagus, stomach, intestines

4. What is the name of the membrane that lines the walls of the abdominopelvic cavity?
   a. Pericardium
   b. Pleural serous membrane
   c. Parietal peritoneum
   d. Visceral peritoneum

5. What is another name for lips?
   a. Labia
   b. Uvula
   c. Frenulum
   d. Dentes

6. Which of the following enzymes breaks down carbohydrates in the mouth?
   a. Lingual lipase
   b. Salivary amylase
   c. Pancreatic lipase
   d. Gastric amylase

7. Where are gastric pits found?
   a. In the lining of the esophagus
   b. In the lining of the pharynx
   c. In the lining of the stomach
   d. In the lining of the small intestine

8. What does the enzyme pepsin break down?
   a. Carbohydrates
   b. Lipids
   c. Proteins
   d. Fats

9. Which enzyme is only found in the stomach of infants?
   a. Gastric lipase
   b. Pepsin
   c. Trypsin
   d. Rennin

10. Which digestive organ is also considered an endocrine gland?
    a. Pancreas
    b. Liver
    c. Gall bladder
    d. Thymus

11. Which of the following are all enzymes found in pancreatic juice?
    a. Trypsin, rennin, pepsin
    b. Pancreatic amylase, trypsin, pancreatic lipase
    c. Salivary amylase, lingual lipase, pepsin
    d. Pancreatic amylase, pepsin, pancreatic lipase

12. Which of the following is a function of the liver?
    a. Carbohydrate metabolism
    b. Protein metabolism
    c. Detoxification
    d. All of the above

13. Where is bile stored?
    a. Liver
    b. Gall bladder
    c. Duodenum
    d. Bile ducts

14. Which of the following are all parts of the small intestine?
    a. Ascending colon, jejunum, anus
    b. Duodenum, jejunum, cecum
    c. Duodenum, jejunum, ileum
    d. Ascending colon, jejunum, rectum

15. Where does approximately 90% of all digestion take place?
    a. Stomach
    b. Small intestine
    c. Large intestine
    d. Colon

12 The Urinary System

Review/Self–Study Notes

1. The kidney's function in cleaning the blood is well known; however, these vital organs play many other important roles in the body. The functions of the kidneys are listed below. Explain each of them in your own words.

   • Regulation of blood composition and volume _____

   _____

   _____

   _____

   • Regulation of blood pH _____

   _____

   _____

   _____

   • Regulation of blood pressure _____

   _____

   _____

   _____

   • Synthesis of calcitriol _____

   _____

   _____

   _____

   • Secretion of erythropoietin _____

   _____

   _____

   _____

- Synthesis of glucose _____

_____

_____

_____

2. The diagram below shows the internal structure of a kidney. Color and label it.

KEY: THE KIDNEY		
Structure	Function/Description	Color
Adrenal gland		
Renal artery and vein		
Renal capsule		
Renal cortex		
Renal column		
Pyramid in renal medulla		
Renal pelvis		
Ureter		
Renal sinus		
Minor calyx		
Major calyx		

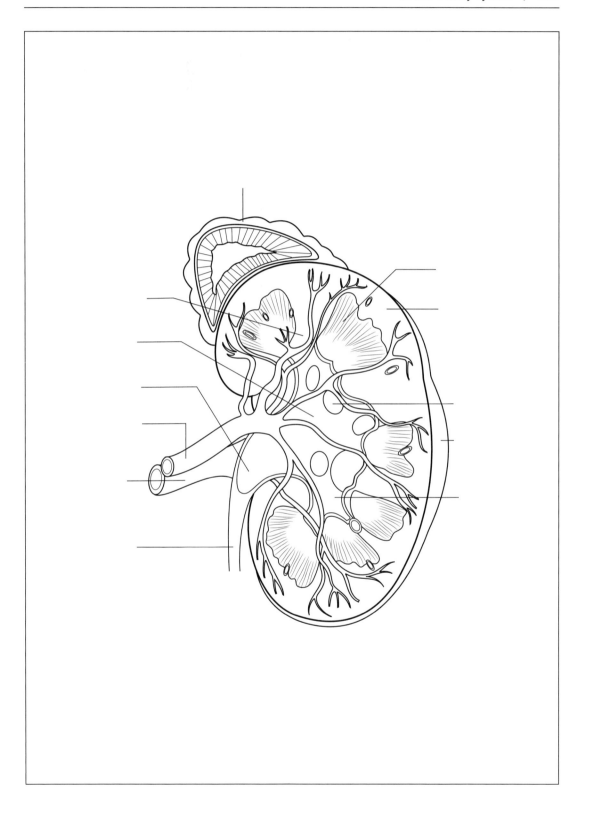

3. Nephrons are the functional units of the kidneys, and it is here that urine is produced and that the volume and composition of blood are regulated. To help you understand how this happens, create a spider diagram or mind map that follows the route of blood through the nephron and the production of urine within the nephron. Ensure you include the following:
   - Renal corpuscle—glomerular filtration:
     - Glomerulus
     - Glomerular capsule
     - Afferent arteriole
     - Efferent arteriole
     - Filtration membrane
   - Renal tubule—tubular secretion and reabsorption:
     - Proximal convoluted tubule
     - Loop of Henle
     - Distal convoluted tubule

4. The kidneys excrete approximately 1¾–3½ pints (1–2 liters) of urine a day. Complete the table below, which lists the solutes present in the normal urine of a healthy person.

Solute	Description
Urea	
Creatinine	
Uric acid	
Urobilinogen	
Inorganic ions	

5. There are a number of different hormones that are all associated with the functioning of the kidneys. Explain the role each of these hormones plays and beneath your explanation write a mnemonic or draw a symbol that will remind you of this hormone's function.

- Parathyroid hormone _____

_____

Mnemonic: _____

_____

- Calcitonin _____

_____

Mnemonic: _____

_____

- Aldosterone _____

_____

Mnemonic: _____

_____

- Renin _____

_____

Mnemonic: _____

_____

- Antidiuretic hormone (vasopressin) _____

_____

Mnemonic: _____

_____

6. Once you have mastered the kidneys, the remaining structures of the urinary system are quite straightforward. However, it is easy to confuse the ureters with the urethra, so write a short sentence describing each of the following.

- Ureters _____

_____

- Bladder _____

_____

- Urethra _____

_____

7. Color and label the diagram of the urinary system below.

KEY: THE URINARY SYSTEM		
Structure	**Function/Description**	**Color**
Kidney		
Ureter		
Bladder		
Urethra		

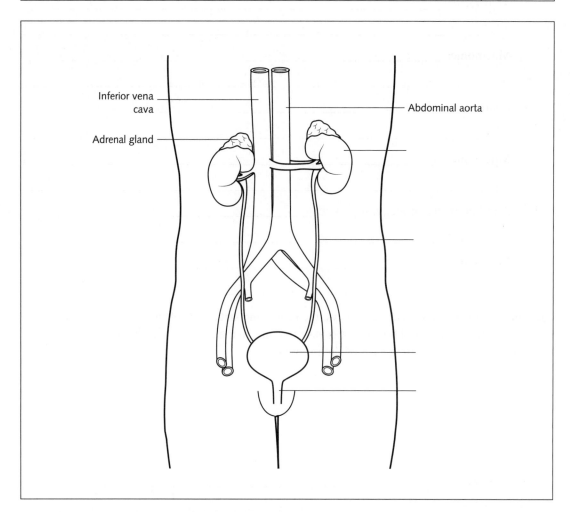

Common pathologies of the urinary system

8. List the common "red-flag" urinary signs and symptoms that should be referred to a doctor for further investigation:

    - _____

    - _____

    - _____

    - _____

    - _____

9. Write down a short phrase that will remind you of each of the following diseases and disorders.

    - Calculi _____

    - Enuresis _____

    - Nephritis (Bright's disease) _____

    - Nephroblastoma (Wilms' tumor) _____

    - Pyelitis _____

    - Renal failure _____

    - Uremia _____

    - Urinary incontinence _____

    - Urinary tract infection _____

    - Pyelonephritis _____

    - Ureteritis _____

    - Urethritis _____

    - Cystitis _____

Exercises

1. The kidneys have many vital functions in the body and some of these have been listed and explained in the table below. Match the correct explanation to its function and write your answers in the spaces below.

Function	Explanation of Function
1. Regulation of blood composition and volume	a. The kidneys help synthesize the active form of vitamin D
2. Regulation of blood pH	b. The kidneys secrete a hormone that stimulates the production of red blood cells
3. Regulation of blood pressure	c. During periods of starvation the kidneys function in gluconeogenesis
4. Synthesis of calcitriol	d. The kidneys filter out and excrete differing amounts of hydrogen ions from the blood
5. Synthesis of erythropoietin	e. The kidneys secrete an enzyme called renin, which causes an increase in blood volume and pressure
6. Synthesis of glucose	f. The kidneys filter blood, remove from it any substances that are no longer needed, and restore certain amounts of water and solutes to the blood as needed

Answers:

1. _____ 2. _____ 3. _____ 4. _____ 5. _____ 6. _____

2. Fill in the missing words in the spaces below.

a. The kidneys are uniquely structured to filter _____ and produce

_____.

b. Above each kidney sits an _____ gland.

c. If you cut a kidney lengthwise you will see that it has three distinct regions: the

outer renal _____, the middle renal _____ and the inner renal

_____.

d. The functional units of the kidney, where urine is formed, are called _____.

3. Once urine has formed in the nephron, it drains through a series of structures before it is excreted from the body. The flow chart below shows this flow of urine, but it is incorrect. Put it into the correct order.

Flow of urine

a. Nephron
⇓
b. Urethra
⇓
c. External environment
⇓
d. Minor calyx
⇓
e. Bladder
⇓
f. Papillary duct
⇓
g. Renal pelvis
⇓
h. Major calyx
⇓
i. Ureter

Answers:

1. _____

2. _____

3. _____

4. _____

5. _____

6. _____

7. _____

8. _____

9. _____

4. Nephrons filter blood through the process of glomerular filtration. The figure below shows a nephron with its associated blood vessels. Label this diagram.

a. _____ b. _____ c. _____ d. _____

_____ _____ _____

j. _____

i. _____

h. _____

g. _____

e. _____

f. _____

5. Below is a list of substances that can be found in urine. Cross out all those that are not normally found in the urine of a healthy person.
   - Hemoglobin
   - Creatinine
   - Pus
   - Uric acid
   - Inorganic ions
   - Glucose
   - Urobilinogen
   - Proteins
   - Red blood cells
   - Bile pigments
   - Urea

6. **Are the following statements true or false? Write T or F in the spaces provided.**

   a. Intracellular fluid is the fluid inside cells. _____

   b. Blood plasma, cerebrospinal fluid, serous fluid, and lymph are all examples of intracellular fluid. _____

   c. Water functions as a solvent in the body. _____

   d. The small tube leading from the bladder to the external environment is called a ureter.

   _____

   e. Females have smaller bladders than males. _____

Common pathologies of the urinary system

7. **In the table below match the disease or disorder to its correct description, and write your answers in the spaces provided.**

Disease/Disorder	Description
1. Calculi	**a.** Abnormal or unusual bed-wetting
2. Enuresis	**b.** The kidney's inability to filter blood efficiently
3. Nephritis	**c.** The involuntary passing of urine
4. Renal failure	**d.** Inflammation of the kidneys
5. Urinary incontinence	**e.** Hard masses that form in the urinary tract; commonly called kidney, bladder, or ureteral stones

   Answers:

   1. _____   2. _____   3. _____   4. _____   5. _____

Vocabulary test

Complete the table below.

WORD	DEFINITION
1. _____	Excretion of more than three liters of urine per day
2. _____	Painful or uncomfortable urination
3. _____	The presence of protein in the urine
4. _____	The presence of red blood cells in the urine
5. _____	Failure of the kidneys to produce urine
6. _____	The production of unusually small amounts of urine
7. _____	The need to urinate regularly during the night

Multiple-Choice Questions

1. **Which of the following are all functions of the kidneys?**
   a. Thermogenesis, regulation of blood pressure, synthesis of erythropoietin
   b. Regulation of blood composition and volume, regulation of blood pH, synthesis of calcitriol
   c. Regulation of blood pressure, synthesis of glucose, desquamation
   d. Regulation of blood pH, thermogenesis, deglutition

2. **What is the name of the outer region of a kidney?**
   a. Renal cortex
   b. Renal medulla
   c. Renal pelvis
   d. Renal sinus

3. **Where in a kidney is urine formed?**
   a. Hilus
   b. Calyx
   c. Nephron
   d. Pelvis

4. **Where inside a nephron do the processes of secretion and reabsorption take place?**
   a. Glomerulus
   b. Afferent arteriole
   c. Renal corpuscle
   d. Renal tubule

5. **What is the name of the closed end of the renal tubule?**
   a. Glomerulus
   b. Glomerular capsule
   c. Loop of Henle
   d. Convoluted tubule

6. **Where in the renal tubule does the reabsorption of the majority of substances occur?**
   a. Proximal convoluted tubule
   b. Loop of Henle
   c. Distal convoluted tubule
   d. Glomerulus

7. **Where in the renal tubule does the "fine-tuning" of the filtrate occur?**
   a. Proximal convoluted tubule
   b. Loop of Henle
   c. Distal convoluted tubule
   d. Glomerulus

8. **What is the name of the vessels that bring blood to the kidneys?**
   a. Hepatic portal veins
   b. Hepatic arteries
   c. Renal veins
   d. Renal arteries

9. **Which of the following statements is correct?**
   a. Efferent arterioles bring blood to the glomerulus and afferent arterioles drain blood from the glomerulus
   b. Afferent arterioles bring blood to the glomerulus and efferent arterioles drain blood from the glomerulus
   c. Peritubular arterioles bring blood to the glomerulus and peritubular venules drain blood from the glomerulus
   d. Peritubular venules bring blood to the glomerulus and peritubular arterioles drain blood from the glomerulus

10. Which of the following solutes are all normal in the urine of a healthy person?
    a. Urea, uric acid, inorganic ions
    b. Glucose, proteins, red blood cells
    c. Pus, proteins, urea
    d. Hemoglobin, uric acid, red blood cells

11. Which of the following hormones all play a role in regulating tubular reabsorption?
    a. Thyroid hormone, progesterone, calcitonin
    b. Antidiuretic hormone (vasopressin), melanocyte-stimulating hormone, estrogen
    c. Parathyroid hormone, aldosterone, calcitonin
    d. Antidiuretic hormone (vasopressin), prolactin, estrogen

12. Which of the following is not an electrolyte?
    a. Calcium
    b. Melatonin
    c. Potassium
    d. Sodium

13. What is a diuretic?
    a. A substance that stimulates an increase in urine production
    b. A substance that stimulates a decrease in urine production
    c. A substance that stimulates an increase in blood pressure
    d. A substance that stimulates a decrease in blood pressure

14. What is the name of the passageway that functions in discharging urine from the body?
    a. Ureter
    b. Bladder
    c. Urethra
    d. Collecting tubule

15. If a person is suffering from fluid retention and blood in the urine, which of the following disorders could they have?
    a. Incontinence
    b. Nephritis
    c. Enuresis
    d. Nocturia

13 The Reproductive System

Review/Self–Study Notes

1. Reproduction is the process by which a new member of a species is produced and reproductive cell division occurs through a process called meiosis. However, meiosis is often confused with mitosis, so, putting yourself into the examiner's position, make up four questions on these processes. Once you have written down these questions, see if you can answer them.

- Question 1: _____

  Answer: _____

  _____

  _____

  _____

- Question 2: _____

  Answer: _____

  _____

  _____

  _____

- Question 3: _____

  Answer: _____

  _____

  _____

  _____

- Question 4: _____

  Answer: _____

  _____

  _____

  _____

2. The diagram below is an overview of the male urinary and genital systems. Color and label it.

KEY: THE MALE URINARY AND GENITAL SYSTEMS		
Structure	**Function/Description**	**Color**
Mid-sagittal view		
Testis		
Epididymis		
Scrotal sac		
Vas deferens		
Seminal vesicle		
Ejaculatory duct		
Prostate gland		
Prostatic urethra		
Bulbourethral (Cowper's) gland		
Bulb of penis		
Spongy urethra		
External urethral orifice		
Ureter		
Bladder		
Urethral sphincter		
Penis		
Glans penis		
Prepuce (foreskin)		

Sacrum

Rectum

Pubic symphysis

3. The diagrams below show the female urinary and genital systems. Color and label them.

KEY: THE FEMALE URINARY AND GENITAL SYSTEMS		
Structure	Function/Description	Color
Mid-sagittal view		
Ovary		
Fallopian tube		
Uterus		
Cervix		
Vagina		
Vulva (clitoris, vestibule, labium minus, labium majus)		
Mons pubis		
Ureter		
Bladder		
Urethra		

Sacrum

Rectum

Pubic symphysis

KEY: THE FEMALE URINARY AND GENITAL SYSTEMS		
Structure	Function/Description	Color
Anterior view		
Ovary		
Ligament of ovary		
Fallopian tube		
Body of uterus		
Uterine fundus		
Uterine cavity		
Uterine cervix		
Cervical canal		
External os		
Vagina		
Endometrium		
Myometrium		
Perimetrium		
Broad ligament		

Suspensory
ligament

Ureter

Uterosacral ligament

4. The diagram below shows the female mammary gland. Color and label it.

KEY: THE MAMMARY GLAND		
Structure	**Function/Description**	**Color**
Adipose tissue		
Glandular tissue		
Lobule containing alveolar glands		
Mammary duct		
Lactiferous duct		

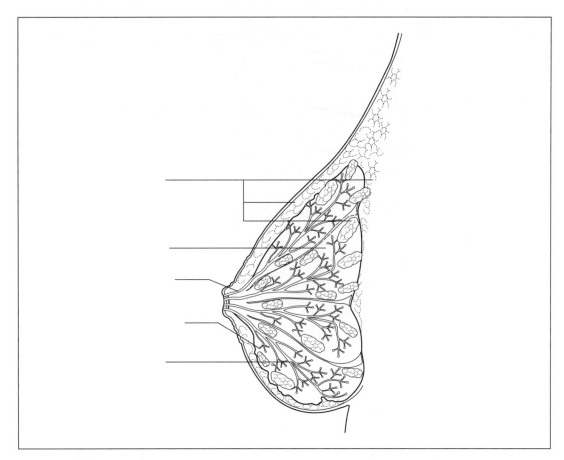

5. **To help you understand the female reproductive cycle, draw a spider diagram or mind map that describes the following phases. The first phase has been started for you.**
   - Menstrual phase
   - Preovulatory phase
   - Ovulation
   - Postovulatory phase

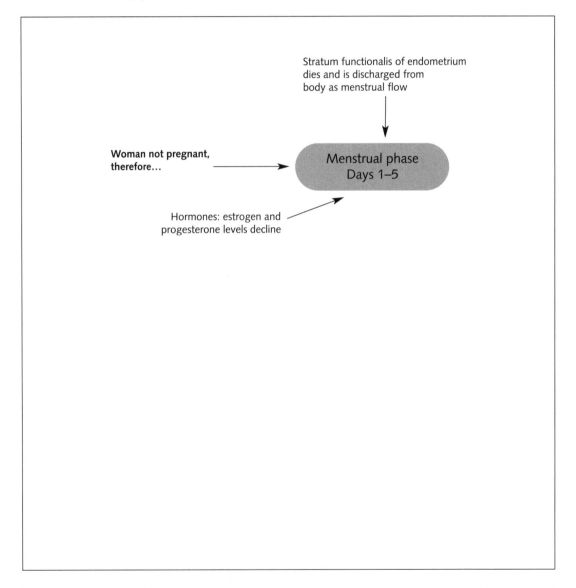

Study tip

Use color and images to make your spider diagram or mind map as personal, fun, and interesting as possible. That way you will find it easier to remember the facts!

6. Use a few memorable words or a short phrase to describe each of the following phases.

- Puberty _____

- Pregnancy _____

- Menopause _____

Common pathologies of the reproductive system

7. Write down a short phrase that will remind you of each of the following diseases and disorders.

Diseases and disorders of the male reproductive system:

- Benign prostatic hyperplasia (BPH)

  _____

- Epididymitis _____

- Impotence _____

- Penile cancer _____

- Prostate cancer _____

- Prostatitis _____

- Testicular cancer _____

Diseases and disorders of the female reproductive system:

- Breast cancer _____

- Cervical cancer _____

- Ectopic pregnancy _____

- Endometriosis _____

- Fibroids _____

- Infertility _____

- Mastitis _____

- Amenorrhea _____

- Dysmenorrhea _____

- Menorrhagia _____

- Premenstrual syndrome _____

- Pelvic inflammatory disease (PID)

  _____

- Polycystic ovary syndrome (Stein-Leventhal syndrome) _____

  _____

- Postnatal depression _____

- Prolapsed uterus _____

- Pre-eclampsia _____

- Toxic shock syndrome _____

- Vaginitis _____

Sexually transmitted infections:

- Chlamydia _____

- Gonorrhea _____

- Human papillomavirus (HPV) infection _____

- Syphilis _____

- Trichomoniasis _____

Exercises

1. Define the words meiosis and mitosis.

   a. Meiosis is _____

   _____

   _____

   b. Mitosis is _____

   _____

   _____

2. Complete the table below, which highlights the differences between meiosis and mitosis.

Characteristic	Meiosis	Mitosis
Number of daughter cells produced	a.	b.
Are daughter cells identical?	c.	d.
Number of chromosomes in each daughter cell	e.	f.

3. Connect the organs and structures below to where they belong.

Scrotum   Penis   Vulva

Ovaries

Vas deferens

Epididymis   Testes

Uterus

Male   Female

Vagina

Seminal vesicles

Spermatic cord   Bulbourethral glands

Prostate   Mammary glands   Fallopian tubes

4. **Are the following statements true or false? Write T or F in the spaces provided.**

   a. The testes are the gonads of the female reproductive system. _____

   b. The testes produce sperm through the process of spermatogenesis. _____

   c. The testes also produce sex hormones called estrogens, which stimulate the development of masculine secondary sex characteristics. _____

   d. The journey of sperm from the testes into the penis is as follows: formed in the seminiferous tubules of the testes → travel down the epididymis, where they mature → into the vas deferens → into the spermatic cord → the spermatic cord takes the sperm into the penis, where they become semen. _____

   e. The function of the penis is to excrete urine and ejaculate semen. _____

5. **Use the clues given to unjumble the letters below.**

   a. AENSTNMIRUOT _____

   b. TOECOY _____

   c. PFAOEIUALSBTLN _____

   d. EMIDNRTMOEU _____

   e. TMPURUUCSOEL _____

   f. LIAOAAIELGCNFRFL _____

   Clues:
   - An immature ovum
   - A large fluid-filled follicle that ruptures to expel an ovum during ovulation
   - After ovulation this empty follicle develops into a glandular structure that produces female hormones
   - Two thin tubes running from the ovaries to the uterus
   - The tissue that lines the inside of the uterus
   - The process by which the lining of the uterus is shed and discarded

6. **Below you will find three descriptions of the female reproductive cycle. Which description is correct?**

   a. Menstruation normally lasts approximately five days and the last day of menstruation is termed day 1 of a woman's cycle. Before it begins, a woman's uterus is not yet prepared to receive a fertilized ovum. If it does not receive a fertilized ovum, the levels of estrogens and progesterone increase and the stratum functionalis dies and is discharged from the body via menstrual flow. After menstruation, a mature Graafian follicle forms and the endometrium proliferates until around day 3 of a 28-day cycle, when the Graafian follicle ruptures to release an ovum into the pelvic cavity. This is called ovulation, and is the time in which a woman can become pregnant. For approximately three days after ovulation the endometrium awaits the arrival of a fertilized ovum. The endometrium is now thickened, highly vascularized, and secreting tissue fluid and glycogen. If fertilization has occurred, a woman will become pregnant. If it has not occurred, menstruation and the reproductive cycle begin again.

b. Menstruation normally lasts approximately five days and the first day of menstruation is termed day 1 of a woman's cycle. Before it begins, a woman's uterus is prepared to receive a fertilized ovum. If it does not receive a fertilized ovum, the levels of estrogens and progesterone decline and the stratum functionalis dies and is discharged from the body via menstrual flow. After menstruation, a mature Graafian follicle forms and the endometrium proliferates until around day 14 of a 28-day cycle, when the Graafian follicle ruptures to release an ovum into the pelvic cavity. This is called ovulation and is the time in which a woman can become pregnant. For approximately 14 days after ovulation the endometrium awaits the arrival of a fertilized ovum. The endometrium is now thickened, highly vascularized, and secreting tissue fluid and glycogen. If fertilization has occurred, a woman will become pregnant. If it has not occurred, menstruation and the reproductive cycle begin again.

c. Menstruation normally lasts approximately ten days and the first day of menstruation is termed day 1 of a woman's cycle. Before it begins, a woman's uterus is prepared to receive a fertilized ovum. If it does not receive a fertilized ovum, the levels of androgens and testosterone decline and the stratum functionalis dies and is discharged from the body via menstrual flow. After menstruation, a mature sperm forms and the endometrium proliferates until around day 14 of a 28-day cycle, when the Graafian follicle ruptures to release a sperm into the pelvic cavity. This is called fertilization and is the time in which a woman can become pregnant. For approximately 14 days after ovulation the endometrium awaits the arrival of a fertilized ovum. The endometrium is now thickened, highly vascularized, and secreting tissue fluid and glycogen. If fertilization has occurred, a woman will become pregnant. If it has not occurred, menstruation and the reproductive cycle begin again.

Answer: _____

Common pathologies of the reproductive system

7. Identify the diseases and disorders below.

a. Inflammation of the prostate gland; symptoms include lower back pain, the urge to

urinate frequently, and burning or painful urination _____

b. A pregnancy in which the fetus develops outside of the uterus _____

c. Inflammation of the breast _____

    d. The absence of a menstrual period _____

    e. A hormonal disorder in which follicles fail to ovulate and instead collect as cysts over

       the ovaries; signs can include acne, weight gain, and irregular vaginal bleeding _____

8. **Circle the signs and symptoms below that should NOT be referred to a doctor for further investigation:**
   a. Solid, painless breast lump
   b. Thickening and dimpling of breast tissue so that it resembles "orange peel"
   c. Discharge of milk from the breast in the mother of a newborn child
   d. Eczema of the nipple or areola
   e. Regular bleeding or purulent discharge from the nipple
   f. Vaginal bleeding accompanied by fever, chills, nausea, and fainting
   g. Vaginal bleeding every 28 days in a 36-year-old woman
   h. Vaginal bleeding after menopause
   i. Blood in the semen for more than one month
   j. Erectile dysfunction accompanied by numbness or paresthesia in the groin/saddle area

9. **In the table below match the hormone to its correct description and write your answers in the spaces provided.**

1. Luteinizing hormone (LH)	**a.** Necessary for female reproductive and sexual development
2. Relaxin	**b.** Prepares the body for pregnancy and the breasts for lactation
3. Inhibin	**c.** Increases bone and muscle strength as well as sexual desire
4. Estrogens	**d.** Stimulates ovarian follicles to grow
5. Follicle-stimulating hormone (FSH)	**e.** Stimulates rupture of the mature Graafian follicle and development of the corpus luteum
6. Progesterone	**f.** Inhibits secretion of FSH
7. Testosterone	**g.** Helps prepare a pregnant woman's body for childbirth

Answers:
1. _____ 2. _____ 3. _____ 4. _____ 5. _____ 6. _____ 7. _____

Vocabulary test

Complete the table below.

WORD	DEFINITION
a. _____	The union and fusion of an ovum and a spermatozoon to form a zygote
b. _____	A cell with a single set of chromosomes
c. _____	The secretion of milk by the mammary glands
d. _____	The production of mature ova in the ovaries
e. _____	Fluid containing sperm and a mixture of fluids secreted by the reproductive glands

Multiple-Choice Questions

1. What is the name given to the process in which a reproductive cell divides to produce four daughter cells, each with only 23 chromosomes?
   a. Mitosis
   b. Meiosis
   c. Oogenesis
   d. Spermatogenesis

2. Which of the following structures is found in both male and female bodies?
   a. Scrotum
   b. Uterus
   c. Urethra
   d. Testes

3. What is the function of the testes?
   a. Mitosis
   b. Meiosis
   c. Oogenesis
   d. Spermatogenesis

4. In which of the following structures do sperm mature?
   a. Epididymis
   b. Vas deferens
   c. Spermatic cord
   d. Urethra

5. Which of the following structures all secrete fluids that combine with sperm to form semen?
   a. Seminal vesicles, mammary glands, bulbourethral glands
   b. Prostate gland, corpus luteum, Graafian follicle
   c. Bulbourethral glands, prostate gland, seminal vesicles
   d. Mammary glands, corpus luteum, corpus albicans

6. **What is the name of the hormone responsible for the development of masculine secondary sexual characteristics?**
   a. Follicle-stimulating hormone
   b. Estrogen
   c. Progesterone
   d. Testosterone

7. **Where are the ovaries located?**
   a. The inferior portion of the pelvic cavity beneath the uterus
   b. The middle portion of the pelvic cavity inside the uterus
   c. The middle portion of the pelvic cavity below the uterus
   d. The superior portion of the pelvic cavity on either side of the uterus

8. **Which of the following statements is true?**
   a. An ovarian follicle enlarges to become a Graafian follicle, which ruptures to expel an oocyte in the process of ovulation
   b. An ovarian follicle enlarges to become the corpus luteum, which ruptures to expel an oocyte in the process of ovulation
   c. An ovarian follicle enlarges to become a Graafian follicle, which ruptures to expel a mature ovum in the process of ovulation
   d. An ovarian follicle enlarges to become the corpus luteum, which ruptures to expel a mature ovum in the process of ovulation

9. **Where in the female reproductive system do the sperm and ovum unite and fuse to form a zygote?**
   a. Urethra
   b. Fallopian tubes
   c. Uterus
   d. Ovaries

10. **What is the name of the layer of tissue that lines the uterus and is shed during menstruation?**
    a. Stratum functionalis
    b. Stratum basalis
    c. Perimetrium
    d. Myometrium

11. **What is the name of the principal hormone that stimulates the production of milk in the mammary glands?**
    a. Luteinizing hormone
    b. Relaxin
    c. Inhibin
    d. Prolactin

12. **How long is an average pregnancy?**
    a. One trimester
    b. Two trimesters
    c. Three trimesters
    d. Four trimesters

13. **What are the female gonads called?**
    a. Ovaries
    b. Oocytes
    c. Ova
    d. Gametes

14. **What is the name of a specialist who deals with the female reproductive system?**
    a. Oncologist
    b. Gynecologist
    c. Urologist
    d. Hematologist

15. **What is the name of the disorder in which endometrial tissue develops outside of the uterus?**
    a. Benign prostatic hyperplasia
    b. Endometriosis
    c. Fibroids
    d. Mastitis

PART 2

Practice Quizzes

Practice Quiz 1

1. A plane that divides the body into upper and lower portions is:
   a. Transverse
   b. Sagittal
   c. Oblique
   d. Frontal (coronal)

2. The stomach is found mainly in:
   a. Right upper quadrant
   b. Left upper quadrant
   c. Right lower quadrant
   d. Left lower quadrant

3. The integumentary system comprises:
   a. Lymph glands, antibodies, and spleen
   b. Stomach, spleen, and liver
   c. Heart, lungs, and blood
   d. Skin, hair, and nails

4. The dermis is made up of:
   a. Epithelial tissues only
   b. Connective tissues only
   c. Epithelial and connective tissues
   d. Neither epithelial nor connective tissues

5. Which cells are present in the stratum basale (germinativum)?
   a. Melanocytes
   b. Merkel cells
   c. Langerhans cells
   d. All of the above

6. Mature bone cells are known as:
   a. Osteoblasts
   b. Adipocytes
   c. Osteocytes
   d. Fibroblasts

7. There are _____ phalanges in the human body.
   a. 14
   b. 28
   c. 56
   d. 60

8. Visceral muscle is:
   a. Found in the walls of the heart
   b. Under the control of the will
   c. Striped in appearance
   d. Found in the walls of hollow organs

9. Fascicles are:
   a. Groups of tendons
   b. Bundles of fascia
   c. Bundles of muscle fibers
   d. Actin filaments

10. What is lacking when ATP is made anaerobically?
    a. Calcium
    b. Oxygen
    c. Lactic acid
    d. ADP

11. The cranial nerves are:
    a. Always sensory
    b. Always motor
    c. May be mixed
    d. Are never mixed

12. A nerve impulse is known as a/an:
    a. Synapse
    b. Action potential
    c. Node of Ranvier
    d. Neurotransmitter

13. The outer layer of the meninges, continuous with the periosteum of the cranium, is the:
    a. Dura mater
    b. Arachnoid mater
    c. Cranial mater
    d. Pia mater

14. Hormones bind to receptors located on:
    a. Brain cells
    b. All cells
    c. Target cells
    d. Gland cells

15. Which of the following is a true statement regarding the endocrine system?
    a. The adrenal cortex is essential to life
    b. The thyroid is essential to life
    c. The ovaries are essential to life
    d. The testes are essential to life

16. Which of the following statements is correct?
    a. Hypersecretion of insulin causes diabetes mellitus
    b. Hypersecretion of melatonin causes seasonal affective disorder
    c. Hyposecretion of human growth hormone causes acromegaly
    d. Hyposecretion of oxytocin causes sterility

17. Cilia are:
    a. Tiny glands
    b. Tiny hairs
    c. Tiny nerves
    d. Tiny blood vessels

18. The epiglottis prevents:
    a. Choking
    b. Asthma
    c. Colds
    d. Laryngitis

19. The heart lies in the area of the thorax known as the:
    a. Septum
    b. Epicardium
    c. Myocardium
    d. Mediastinum

20. Which one of the following is a high-pressure system?
    a. Arterial
    b. Venous
    c. Pulmonary
    d. Capillary

21. The digestive system consists of:
    a. The alimentary canal and the gastrointestinal tract
    b. The liver, gall bladder, and pancreas
    c. The gastrointestinal tract only
    d. The alimentary canal, liver, gall bladder, and pancreas

22. Terms that are associated with the urinary system are:
    a. Nephrology
    b. Renal
    c. Both of the above
    d. Neither of the above

23. Which hormone below is not associated with renal function?
    a. Prolactin
    b. Aldosterone
    c. ADH (vasopressin)
    d. Parathormone

24. The uterus is situated:
    a. On the posterior abdominal wall
    b. In front of the bladder and behind the rectum
    c. Behind the bladder and in front of the rectum
    d. On the lateral walls of the pelvis

25. The journey the sperm takes in order to fertilize the ovum is (in the correct order):
    a. Vagina, uterus, ovary, cervix
    b. Fallopian tube, uterus, cervix, vagina
    c. Uterus, vagina, cervix, ovary
    d. Vagina, cervix, uterus, fallopian tube

Practice Quiz 2

1. The thoracic cavity contains the:
   a. Heart, brain, liver
   b. Heart, lungs, esophagus
   c. Brain, liver, lungs
   d. Esophagus, heart, liver

2. The imaginary line down the center of the body is the:
   a. Proximal line
   b. Distal line
   c. Midline
   d. Frontline

3. Hair is found all over the body except:
   a. Eyelids, lips, and tongue
   b. Lips, soles, and palms
   c. Palms, soles, and ears
   d. Palms, lips, and eyelids

4. Cells that have a sensory function in the epidermis are:
   a. Merkel cells
   b. Keratinocytes
   c. Melanocytes
   d. Langerhans cells

5. The process by which cartilage is replaced by bone is called:
   a. Osteology
   b. Ossification
   c. Osteocytology
   d. Osteoporosis

6. The function of a ligament is to:
   a. Connect muscle to bone
   b. Connect tendon to muscle
   c. Connect bone to bone
   d. Connect muscle to muscle

7. Muscles can:
   a. Maintain posture
   b. Move substances within the body
   c. Generate heat
   d. All of the above

8. Tendons and aponeuroses are formed from:
   a. Epimysium
   b. Perimysium
   c. Endomysium
   d. All of the above

9. The integrative function of the nervous system is to:
   a. Detect stimuli from both inside and outside the body
   b. Make decisions regarding information received
   c. Stimulate the endocrine system to act
   d. Enable effectors to maintain homeostasis

10. There are _____ pairs of spinal nerves.
    a. 8
    b. 12
    c. 24
    d. 31

11. Endocrine glands are called "ductless" glands because:
    a. Hormones are secreted directly into the bloodstream
    b. Their ducts connect directly with the bloodstream
    c. The production of hormones is intermittent
    d. They produce hormones

12. Endocrine glands that also have an exocrine function are the:
    a. Pituitary
    b. Pancreas
    c. Sebaceous
    d. Sudoriferous

13. The only organ in the body that can perform gaseous exchange of oxygen and carbon dioxide is:
    a. The skin
    b. The lung
    c. The kidney
    d. The liver

14. The process by which air is drawn in and out of the lungs is:
    a. Ventilation
    b. Internal respiration
    c. Pulmonary respiration
    d. All of these

15. Which list best describes the functions of the cardiovascular system?
    a. Respiration, protection, transportation
    b. Excretion, defense, regulation of temperature
    c. Transportation, protection, excretion
    d. Regulation, transportation, protection

16. Erythrocytes are shaped like biconcave discs because:
    a. They do not have a nucleus
    b. Hemoglobin molecules are also shaped like this

c. The shape ensures a large surface area
    d. The shape enables them to clump together to prevent blood loss

17. The thin, smooth lining of the inside of the heart is the:
    a. Endocardium
    b. Visceral pericardium
    c. Parietal pericardium
    d. Epicardium

18. These structures vary in size from a pinhead to an almond, they filter lymph, and remove or destroy harmful substances.
    a. Lymphatic vessels
    b. Lymphatic ducts
    c. Lymph nodes
    d. Lymphatic capillaries

19. The two lymphatic ducts are:
    a. Right and left lymphatic
    b. Right and left subclavian
    c. Thoracic and right lymphatic
    d. Thoracic and left lymphatic

20. The fingerlike projection hanging down from the soft palate is the:
    a. Labia
    b. Frenulum
    c. Uvula
    d. Papilla

21. The head of the pancreas lies:
    a. Under the liver
    b. In the curve of the duodenum

c. Between the ileum and the jejunum
    d. In the left lower quadrant

22. _____ result(s) from protein breakdown.
    a. Amino acids
    b. Glucose
    c. Fatty acids
    d. Glycogen

23. The kidneys are to be found:
    a. Just below the waist
    b. Between T12 and L3 vertebrae
    c. Attached to the posterior abdominal wall
    d. All of the above

24. Which of the following is true?
    a. The seminal vesicles secrete an acidic fluid that helps to nourish the sperm
    b. Secretions from the prostate gland help to reduce the motility and viability of sperm
    c. Semen is the combined secretions of the prostate, seminal vesicles, and Cowper's glands
    d. Semen is slightly acidic in order to neutralize the environment within the vagina

25. Breastfeeding requires:
    a. Prolactin
    b. Oxytocin
    c. Both of these
    d. Neither of these

Practice Quiz 3

1. The study of disease in the body is:
    a. Physiology
    b. Cytology
    c. Histology
    d. Pathology

2. Cervical refers to the:
    a. Legs
    b. Neck
    c. Arms
    d. Back

3. The skin plays an important part in raising body temperature by:
    a. Vasoconstriction
    b. Sweating
    c. Vasodilation
    d. None of the above

4. This layer of skin is waterproof, has cells with no nuclei, and is most apparent on the palms of the hands and soles of the feet.
    a. Stratum basale (germinativum)
    b. Stratum granulosum
    c. Stratum lucidum
    d. Stratum corneum

5. Haversian systems can be found:
   a. In the long bones only
   b. In compact bone only
   c. In cancellous (spongy) bone only
   d. In both compact and cancellous bone

6. The tibia is commonly known as:
   a. The breastbone
   b. The kneecap
   c. The thigh bone
   d. The shin bone

7. An aponeurosis is:
   a. A large cylindrical ligament
   b. A flat, sheet-like tendon
   c. The plasma membrane of a muscle cell
   d. A contractile element of skeletal muscle

8. This type of muscle has spindle-shaped cells with a single nucleus.
   a. Smooth
   b. Cardiac
   c. Skeletal
   d. All types of muscle

9. Which of the following is not true?
   a. The overall function of the nervous system is to maintain homeostasis
   b. The nervous system works with the endocrine system to maintain homeostasis
   c. The nervous system relies upon hormones to effect change
   d. The endocrine system is regarded as a "slower" system than the nervous system

10. Digestion is under the control of which part of the nervous system?
    a. Peripheral
    b. Central
    c. Somatic
    d. Autonomic

11. The hormones produced by the endocrine system are regulated by:
    a. Positive feedback
    b. Negative feedback
    c. Neither positive nor negative feedback
    d. Both negative and positive feedback

12. Which of the structures below is not situated in the brain?
    a. Parathyroids
    b. Hypothalamus
    c. Posterior pituitary
    d. Anterior pituitary

13. Which of the following are functions of the respiratory system?
    a. Olfaction
    b. Breathing
    c. Producing speech
    d. All of the above

14. Tissue respiration is the same as:
    a. Pulmonary respiration
    b. External respiration
    c. Internal respiration
    d. Cellular respiration

15. Blood is a:
    a. Muscular tissue
    b. Epithelial tissue
    c. Connective tissue
    d. Nervous tissue

16. The wall of the left ventricle is much thicker than the right because:
    a. The left ventricle is much smaller than the right
    b. Blood has to travel a much longer distance
    c. The pressure in the left side is lower than in the right
    d. All of the above

17. Which of the following statements is true regarding the lymphatic system?
    a. Lymph is derived from interstitial fluid and is found only in lymphatic vessels
    b. Lymph has a milky/creamy appearance and is produced by the digestive tract
    c. Lymphatic capillaries are similar to blood capillaries and allow exchange of nutrients
    d. Lymph is derived from the blood and is part of the blood plasma

18. The lymphatic vessels are most like veins in structure because:
    a. They both return their contents to the heart
    b. They both have one-way valves
    c. Their walls are both only one cell thick
    d. Their walls are both thick and muscular

19. Digestion is:
    a. The taking of food and drink into the body
    b. The process by which unwanted food is eliminated from the body
    c. The breaking down of large molecules into smaller ones
    d. The process by which food substances enter the bloodstream

20. Which teeth are used for cutting into food?
    a. Canines
    b. Incisors
    c. Premolars
    d. Molars

21. Which of the following is not a true statement?
    a. More than half the body's weight is made up of water
    b. The body can survive longer without water than without food
    c. Urine is mostly made up of water
    d. The size and shape of every cell is maintained by water

22. The kidneys are protected by:
    a. Adipose tissue
    b. Bones of the pelvis
    c. The vertebral column
    d. All of the above

23. Examples of extracellular fluid are:
    a. Lymph
    b. Interstitial fluid
    c. Cerebrospinal fluid
    d. All of the above

24. Meiosis results in _____ daughter cells.
    a. 4
    b. 2
    c. 2 daughter and 2 son cells
    d. 0

25. The testes:
    a. Lie in the scrotal sac
    b. Produce testosterone
    c. Produce sperm
    d. All of the above

Practice Quiz 4

1. The brain and spinal cord are contained within which body cavity?
    a. Ventral body cavity
    b. Abdominal cavity
    c. Dorsal cavity
    d. Pelvic cavity

2. The hand is _____ to the elbow.
    a. Deep
    b. Distal
    c. Proximal
    d. Superficial

3. Keratinocytes:
    a. Make up 90% of epidermal cells
    b. Produce a pigment to color the skin
    c. Are found only in the stratum basale
    d. Arise from the bone marrow

4. The stage of hair growth that lasts the longest is:
    a. Telogen
    b. Catagen
    c. Anagen
    d. None of the above

5. Which is the only moveable bone in the skull?
    a. Zygomatic
    b. Mandible
    c. Nasal
    d. Maxilla

6. Which of the following joints can permit movement?
    a. Fibrous joints
    b. Coronal sutures
    c. Cartilaginous joints
    d. Synarthrotic joints

7. Which is the heaviest muscle in the human body?
    a. Latissimus dorsi
    b. Gluteus maximus
    c. Teres major
    d. Gastrocnemius

8. The definition of adduct is:
    a. To move toward the midline
    b. To move away from the midline
    c. To bring the soles of the feet together
    d. To make the soles of the feet face outward

9. Dendrites:
    a. Receive information into the cell body
    b. Insulate the axon
    c. Transmit information away from the cell body
    d. Transmit information between sensory and motor neurons

10. The part of the brain that interprets visual images is the:
    a. Frontal lobe
    b. Temporal lobe
    c. Parietal lobe
    d. Occipital lobe

11. Which of these is not caused by abnormal secretion of thyroid hormones?
    a. Cretinism
    b. Tetany
    c. Myxedema
    d. Goiter

12. A "temporary" endocrine gland is the:
    a. Stomach
    b. Placenta
    c. Gall bladder
    d. Urinary bladder

13. The Eustachian tubes open into the:
    a. Nasopharynx
    b. Larynx
    c. Oropharynx
    d. Laryngopharynx

14. The left lung has _____ lobes and the right lung has _____ lobes:
    a. 3 and 2
    b. 1 and 2
    c. 2 and 1
    d. 2 and 3

15. Bradycardia is:
    a. An irregular heart rhythm
    b. A heart rate over 100 beats per minute
    c. A heart rate below 60 beats per minute
    d. None of the above

16. Which of the lists below best describes the functions of the lymphatic system?
    a. Drainage, filtration, immunity, respiration
    b. Immunity, fat transport, production of lymphocytes, respiration
    c. Drainage, fat transport, immunity, filtration
    d. Filtration, immunity, production of lymphocytes, fat transport

17. Inflammation is:
    a. One of the body's responses to injury
    b. Characterized by heat, swelling, redness, and pain
    c. A mechanism to prevent the spread of further tissue damage
    d. All of the above

18. Which of the following statements is false?
    a. The peritoneum, unlike other serous membranes, has only one layer
    b. The peritoneum is the largest serous membrane in the body
    c. The peritoneum is composed of large folds
    d. One of the functions of the peritoneum is to bind organs to the abdominal cavity

19. Obesity can be identified by assessing an individual's _____.
    a. GIT
    b. HCL
    c. BMI
    d. DNA

20. An individual who has intolerance to gluten suffers from _____ disease.
    a. Celiac
    b. Colitis
    c. Crohn's
    d. Colorectal

21. Most reabsorption in the nephron occurs in the:
    a. Bowman's capsule
    b. Collecting duct
    c. Proximal convoluted tubule
    d. All of the above

22. The majority of water in the body is found:
    a. In the blood
    b. Inside the cells
    c. In the digestive system
    d. Outside the cells

23. The uterus is lined with:
    a. Endometrium
    b. Perimetrium
    c. Peritoneum
    d. Myometrium

24. Which one of the following is not a sexually transmitted disease?
    a. Syphilis
    b. Vaginitis
    c. Chlamydia
    d. AIDS

25. Severe postnatal depression is linked to:
    a. Mothers under the age of 20
    b. Mothers over the age of 40
    c. Infection
    d. Hormonal changes

Practice Quiz 5

1. The heart is _____ to the lungs.
    a. Proximal
    b. Lateral
    c. Medial
    d. Distal

2. Which of the following is true regarding lymphatic capillaries?
    a. They are blind (closed)-ended
    b. They are more permeable than blood capillaries
    c. They are not found in the brain
    d. All of the above

3. Examples of effectors are:
    a. Special senses
    b. Cranial nerves
    c. Muscles and glands
    d. Brain and spinal cord

4. Cholecystitis is:
    a. Inflammation of the stomach
    b. Inflammation of the gall bladder
    c. Inflammation of the liver
    d. Inflammation of the pancreas

5. The endocrine system maintains homeostasis with the nervous system but:
    a. Its effects are not as immediate
    b. Its effects are longer lasting
    c. The systems control each other
    d. All of the above

6. The functional units of the kidney are the:
    a. Columns
    b. Calyces
    c. Nephrons
    d. Pyramids

7. Which of the following contain the protein hemoglobin?
    a. Leucocytes
    b. Erythrocytes
    c. Monocytes
    d. Thrombocytes

8. Which of the following is a false statement?
    a. A zygote contains 46 chromosomes
    b. A zygote develops into a new organism
    c. Zygotes continue to divide by meiosis
    d. Zygotes result from fertilization

9. Which of the following is the odd one out?
    a. Occipital
    b. Temporal
    c. Parietal
    d. Lacrimal

10. The liver receives nutrient-rich, deoxygenated blood from the digestive organs via the:
    a. Hepatic vein
    b. Hepatic portal vein
    c. Gastric vein
    d. Inferior mesenteric vein

11. The effect of "jet lag" is attributed to disruption of the production of:
    a. Melatonin
    b. Calcitonin
    c. Oxytocin
    d. Thymosin

12. Which of the following statements is incorrect?
    a. Filtration of the blood occurs in the glomerulus
    b. Filtration of the blood results in water and solutes being forced into the renal tubule
    c. The closed end of the renal tubule is called the collecting duct
    d. Blood cells are not filtered into the renal tubule

13. Chemical digestion of carbohydrates starts in the:
    a. Stomach
    b. Small intestine
    c. Mouth
    d. Large intestine

14. What is meant by atherosclerosis?
    a. Abnormal constriction of the walls of arterioles in the fingers and toes
    b. Inflammation of the walls of veins
    c. Enlarged and dilated veins in the walls of the rectum and anus
    d. A build-up of fatty substances on the walls of the arteries

15. Pulmonary refers to:
    a. Blood
    b. Nose
    c. Lung
    d. Heart

16. A drug or substance that stimulates an increase in urine production is called:
    a. Antibiotic
    b. Analgesic
    c. Hypnotic
    d. Diuretic

17. The spermatic cord contains:
    a. Urethra, penis, foreskin
    b. Blood and lymphatic vessels, nerves, muscles
    c. Prostate gland, seminal vesicles, bulbourethral glands
    d. Broad ligament, Graafian follicle, corpus luteum

18. The femoral artery can be found in the region of the:
    a. Ankle
    b. Sole
    c. Thigh
    d. Knee

19. The nose is lined with:
    a. Cancellous (spongy) bone
    b. Ciliated mucous membrane
    c. Serous membrane
    d. Yellow elastic tissue

20. Anabolism (protein synthesis) is stimulated by:
    a. Androgens and estrogen
    b. Androgens only
    c. Testosterone only
    d. Progesterone

21. A high-fiber diet can help to prevent:
    a. Ulcers
    b. Jaundice
    c. Constipation
    d. Diarrhea

22. Varicose veins:
    a. May be a contraindication to massage
    b. May be an inherited condition
    c. May be caused by inefficient valves
    d. All of the above

23. In external respiration the blood loses _____.
    a. Oxygen
    b. Nitrogen
    c. Nothing
    d. Carbon dioxide

24. Prolonged hyperventilation can lead to:
    a. Pneumonia
    b. Unconsciousness
    c. A runny nose
    d. All of the above

25. Which endocrine gland is also part of the immune system?
    a. Thyroid
    b. Adrenal cortex
    c. Thymus
    d. Adrenal medulla

26. Lipids and lipid-soluble vitamins are absorbed into the:
    a. Liver
    b. Blood capillaries
    c. Lymph nodes
    d. Lacteals

27. The thenar eminence is found:
    a. On the forehead
    b. At the base of the big toe
    c. At the base of the thumb
    d. At the base of the spine

28. Cartilage, tendons, ligaments, and bone are all examples of:
    a. Connective tissue
    b. Nervous tissue
    c. Muscle tissue
    d. Epithelial tissue

29. Apoptosis is:
    a. A form of mitosis
    b. The process during which cells die
    c. A form of meiosis
    d. The pathological destruction of cells

30. An itchy rash in a specific area resulting from direct contact with cosmetics, metals, or household chemicals could be:
    a. Urticaria (nettle rash or hives)
    b. Eczema

c. Contact dermatitis
d. Folliculitis

31. Carbon dioxide is transported by blood mainly in the:
a. White cells
b. Hemoglobin
c. Plasma
d. Red cells

32. When a muscle contracts but does not shorten and no movement results it is:
a. Isometric contraction
b. Isotonic contraction
c. Eccentric contraction
d. Concentric contraction

33. Mastitis is:
a. More common around the time of childbirth
b. Relieved by massage
c. Inflammation of the vagina
d. A yeast infection

34. Helper T cells aid:
a. The cell-mediated immune response
b. The antibody-mediated immune response
c. Neither immune response
d. Both immune responses

35. Which bone supports the tongue and provides attachment for muscles of the neck and pharynx?
a. Hamate
b. Hyoid
c. Humerus
d. Hyaline

36. Which part of the nervous system is regarded as conserving energy?
a. Central nervous system
b. Peripheral nervous system
c. Sympathetic nervous system
d. Parasympathetic nervous system

37. The technical terms "onyx" and "unguium" refer to:
a. The skin
b. The hair
c. The nails
d. All of the above

38. The term visceral refers to:
a. The inner walls of a body cavity
b. The outer surface of the body
c. The internal organs of the body
d. None of these

39. Anosmia is loss of the sense of:
a. Smell
b. Taste
c. Sight
d. Hearing

40. A basal cell carcinoma may commonly be known as:
a. Melanoma
b. Rodent ulcer
c. Varicose ulcer
d. Squamous cell carcinoma

41. Water makes up about _____ of our bodies.
a. 10%
b. 30%
c. 60%
d. 100%

42. If you push your head backward (while standing upright) to face up to the ceiling, you are:
a. Hypoextending the neck
b. Rotating the neck
c. Hyperextending the neck
d. Circumducting the neck

43. Which is true of stress?
a. Can be good for some people
b. Can be alleviated by complementary therapies
c. Can make people more susceptible to illness and disease
d. All are true

44. The muscular dystrophies:
a. Are infectious conditions
b. Are inherited conditions
c. Are caused by injuries
d. Only occur in women

45. Saliva is _____ in nature.
a. Acidic
b. Alkaline
c. Salty
d. Semi-solid

46. Renal failure:
a. Is a life-threatening condition
b. Could result in having dialysis
c. Could result in having a kidney transplant
d. All of the above

47. Which of the following is a false statement?
a. Some skeletal muscles are not attached to bones
b. Tendons attach skeletal muscles to bones
c. Skeletal muscles are attached to both bones and joints
d. Ligaments attach bones together at joints

48. The body system that contains the largest organ in the body is the:
a. Digestive system
b. Nervous system
c. Integumentary system
d. Immune system

49. Cervical refers to the:
a. Neck
b. Legs
c. Arms
d. Back

50. This muscle's origin includes the occipital bone (back of head) and most of the cervical and thoracic vertebrae; it has upper, middle and lower fibers.
a. Latissimus dorsi
b. Trapezius
c. Deltoid
d. Erector spinae

Practice Quiz 6

1. Which of the following is incorrect with regard to meiosis and mitosis?
   a. Meiosis only occurs in the gonads
   b. Mitosis is essential for growth and repair of cells
   c. Meiosis results in the haploid number
   d. Mitosis ensures genetic diversity

2. Which of these is a false statement regarding the nervous system?
   a. The right cerebral hemisphere controls the right side of the body
   b. The olfactory nerve is a purely sensory nerve
   c. The sciatic nerve is the longest nerve in the body
   d. The meninges cover both the brain and spinal cord

3. Which of the following is not a solute carried by the blood plasma?
   a. Electrolytes
   b. Nutrients
   c. Proteins
   d. pH

4. Prolonged use of a wheelchair or bed rest will result in _____ of the leg muscles.
   a. Hypertrophy
   b. Fatigue
   c. Atrophy
   d. Tonicity

5. In internal respiration, the blood gains _____.
   a. Nutrients
   b. Nitrogen
   c. Carbon dioxide
   d. Oxygen

6. How many teeth does a mature adult have?
   a. 20
   b. 22
   c. 30
   d. 32

7. The main function of the ovary is to:
   a. House the growing fetus
   b. Produce the follicle-stimulating hormone
   c. Produce mature ova
   d. Receive the sperm

8. The five main taste sensations are:
   a. Sweet, sour, bitter, salty, umami
   b. Salty, sweet, spicy, stale, bitter
   c. Bitter, umami, tart, salty, spicy
   d. Sweet, tart, stale, bitter, spicy

9. Collagen and elastin give skin:
   a. Extensibility and strength
   b. Nutrition and hydration
   c. Insulation and shock absorption
   d. Sensitivity and protection

10. The function of mucus within the respiratory system is to:
    a. Exchange gases
    b. Trap impurities
    c. Prevent dehydration
    d. Prevent bleeding

11. Symptoms of premenstrual tension in women include:
    a. Emotional upset
    b. Edema and weight gain
    c. Fatigue and lethargy
    d. All of the above

12. Which of the following is a false statement regarding deep vein thrombosis?
    a. May be caused by inactivity, pregnancy, following surgery
    b. Usually forms in the deep veins of the leg
    c. Is a hereditary disease and runs in families
    d. May become mobile in the bloodstream and cause a pulmonary embolus

13. Muscle cells have many mitochondria because:
    a. Mitochondria are the working units of muscles
    b. All the mitochondria are not always working
    c. Muscle cells use much energy
    d. Muscle cells require much protein

14. Digestion does not take place in:
    a. The mouth
    b. The esophagus
    c. The stomach
    d. The duodenum

15. The function of the spinal cord is:
    a. To connect the brain to the rest of the body
    b. To transmit sensory information from the PNS to the brain
    c. To transmit motor instructions from the brain to the PNS
    d. All of the above

16. Red blood cells do not contain a nucleus because:
    a. They only live for 120 days
    b. Maximum space is required for oxygen transport
    c. They are not able to reproduce
    d. All of the above

17. The alveoli are structured to ensure:
    a. A huge surface area
    b. No friction occurs
    c. Collapsing does not occur
    d. All of the above

18. Which statement is correct?
    a. The penis and clitoris are both made of erectile tissue
    b. The perineum is present in both men and women
    c. The mons pubis protects the symphysis pubis
    d. They are all correct

19. This vitamin is synthesized in the skin:
    a. Vitamin C
    b. Vitamin D
    c. Vitamin E
    d. Vitamin K

20. Which of the following is false?
    a. Cancer sometimes spreads from one site in the body to another
    b. Cancer can be spread via the lymphatic system
    c. Cancer cannot be spread via the bloodstream
    d. It is wise to consider carefully before treating a client who is suffering from cancer

21. Which of the following is a false statement regarding meningitis?
    a. It is inflammation of the meninges
    b. Symptoms can include a headache, stiff neck, or a rash
    c. It can be a fatal disease
    d. The cause is always viral

22. Which muscle flexes, abducts, and laterally rotates the hip joint and flexes the knee joint?
    a. Serratus anterior
    b. Soleus
    c. Sartorius
    d. Supinator

23. Examples of steroid hormones are:
    a. Sex hormones
    b. Oxytocin
    c. Insulin
    d. All of the above

24. How many vertebrae are there in the thoracic (dorsal) spine?
    a. 7
    b. 12
    c. 22
    d. 33

25. If a client reports he has seen blood in his urine he should be advised to:
    a. Drink more water
    b. Visit his doctor
    c. Change his diet
    d. Book in for reflexology

26. The largest single mass of lymphatic tissue in the body is the:
    a. Liver
    b. Adenoids
    c. Tonsils
    d. Spleen

27. Which of the following statements is true regarding tuberculosis?
    a. It is a hospital-acquired infection
    b. It no longer occurs in the Western world
    c. It is caused by an airborne bacterium
    d. All of the above are true

28. The costal cartilages are located:
    a. At the hips
    b. At the neck
    c. At the knee
    d. At the ribs

29. Conception can be prevented by:
    a. Ligation (constriction) of the vas deferens
    b. Manipulation of the hormones by artificial means
    c. Physical barriers to prevent the sperm from reaching the egg
    d. All of the above

30. Which of the following is correct for the order of blood flow?
    a. Body, right side of heart, pulmonary artery, lungs, left side of heart, aorta
    b. Left side of heart, lungs, pulmonary artery, aorta, body, right side of heart
    c. Lungs, right side of heart, body, aorta, left side of heart, pulmonary artery
    d. Right side of heart, pulmonary artery, body, left side of heart, aorta, lungs

31. Which list below would best describe processes coordinated by the endocrine system?
    a. Homeostasis, negative feedback, positive feedback, hormone stimulation
    b. Reproduction, growth, metabolism, homeostasis
    c. Repair, replace, reproduce, restimulate
    d. Hyposecretion, hypersecretion, stimulation, inhibition

32. Which one of the following statements about chloasma is false?
    a. It can occur in pregnant women
    b. It usually affects the forehead, cheeks, and around the lips
    c. It usually fades with time
    d. It is caused by an underproduction of melanin

33. _____ fever is a contagious disease of the lymphatic system common in children and young adults and often called the "kissing" disease.
    a. Rheumatic
    b. Scarlet
    c. Glandular
    d. Yellow

34. Blood and mucus present in the stools may be a sign of:
    a. Colitis
    b. Gingivitis
    c. Cirrhosis
    d. Halitosis

35. Gliding joints are capable of:
    a. Side-to-side and back-and-forth movement
    b. Rotation and circumduction
    c. Adduction and abduction
    d. None of the above

36. The kidneys receive approximately _____ ml of blood per minute.
    a. 12
    b. 120
    c. 1200
    d. 12,000

37. Which of the following is not an epithelial tissue?
    a. Cuboid
    b. Cartilage
    c. Columnar
    d. Ciliated

38. The lymphatic system is part of the:
    a. Digestive system
    b. Cardiovascular system
    c. Immune system
    d. Urinary system

39. Carbohydrate metabolism is affected by:
    a. Cortisol
    b. Progesterone
    c. ADH (vasopressin)
    d. FSH

40. Water is the _____ of all body fluids.
    a. Solution
    b. Solute
    c. Concentrate
    d. Solvent

41. Which of the following statements about simple diffusion is false?
    a. A concentration gradient from high to low is involved
    b. The process continues until equilibrium is reached
    c. The rate of diffusion is affected by temperature
    d. A carrier is needed to help larger substances across the membrane

42. The menopause is characterized by:
    a. Inability to bear children
    b. Cessation of ovulation
    c. Unresponsiveness of the ovaries to FSH
    d. All of the above

43. A painful condition of the joints due to a build-up of uric acid, often found in middle-aged men is:
    a. Bunions
    b. Sprain
    c. Gout
    d. Rickets

44. Dialysis is:
    a. Passing large amounts of urine
    b. Removal of part of a kidney
    c. Mechanical cleansing of the blood
    d. A bacterial infection of the kidney

45. Which statement is false?
    a. Stressed individuals are more likely to suffer from irritable bowel syndrome
    b. "Heartburn" is caused by reflux of acidic stomach contents
    c. Flatulence is bad breath
    d. Hepatitis is inflammation of the liver from a variety of causes

46. Which statement is untrue of hyaline cartilage?
    a. It attaches the ribs to the sternum
    b. It is strong and elastic and found in the external ear
    c. It covers the epiphyses to reduce friction
    d. It allows growth at the epiphyseal plate

47. The layer of hair where pigment granules are found is the:
    a. Cuticle
    b. Matrix
    c. Cortex
    d. Medulla

48. The thorax is superior to the:
    a. Abdomen
    b. Shoulders
    c. Head
    d. Mouth

49. Which is the correct order of the layers of the epidermis from the most superficial to the deepest?
    a. Stratum corneum, stratum germinativum, stratum spinosum, stratum lucidum, stratum granulosum
    b. Stratum germinativum, stratum spinosum, stratum lucidum, stratum granulosum, stratum corneum
    c. Stratum germinativum, stratum spinosum, stratum granulosum, stratum lucidum, stratum corneum
    d. Stratum corneum, stratum lucidum, stratum granulosum, stratum spinosum, stratum germinativum

50. The purpose of the myelin sheath is to:
    a. Enclose the brain and spinal cord
    b. Slow down the transmission of impulses
    c. Wrap around the cell bodies
    d. Speed up transmission of impulses

Practice Quiz 7

1. Blood plasma makes up about _____ of blood:
    a. 35%
    b. 45%
    c. 55%
    d. 65%

2. The gonads are controlled by:
    a. LH and FSH
    b. TSH
    c. GH
    d. MSH and ADH (vasopressin)

3. In an ectopic pregnancy:
    a. The fetus develops too quickly
    b. The fetus develops outside of the uterus

c. The fetus does not develop at all

d. None of the above

4. Lymph transports escaped plasma proteins that cannot return to the blood because:
a. They are too large
b. There are too many of them
c. They are too small
d. Plasma proteins don't escape from the blood

5. The hormones associated with renal function are:
a. Urobilinogen and hemoglobin
b. Urea and rennin
c. Calcitonin and creatinine
d. Erythropoietin and calcitriol

6. The soft, downy hair found over most of the body surface is:
a. Lanugo
b. Follicular
c. Vellus
d. Terminal

7. Which of the following statements is false?
a. The role of neurons is to transmit impulses
b. Neuroglia are smaller and more numerous than neurons
c. Neuroglia insulate, protect, and nurture neurons
d. Both neurons and neuroglia divide by mitosis

8. Which of the following is a false statement regarding skeletal muscle cells?
a. The sarcolemma is the muscle cell membrane
b. Each muscle cell has a nucleus in the center
c. The cytoplasm is called the sarcoplasm
d. A muscle cell is called a muscle fiber

9. Which of the following are salivary glands?
a. Parotid
b. Submandibular

c. Sublingual
d. All of the above

10. Functions of the skeletal system include:
a. Protection, secretion, absorption, movement
b. Muscle attachment, movement, shape, excretion
c. Mineral homeostasis, movement, support, absorption
d. Support, mineral homeostasis, protection, movement

11. Which muscles strengthen and stabilize the shoulder joint?
a. Diaphragm, internal intercostals, external intercostals
b. Erector spinae, latissimus dorsi, trapezius
c. Subscapularis, supraspinatus, infraspinatus, teres minor
d. Teres major, quadratus lumborum, levator scapulae

12. The back of the body is referred to as:
a. Posterior
b. Parietal
c. Proximal
d. Peripheral

13. The ions required for transmission of nerve impulses are:
a. Sodium and chloride
b. Potassium and calcium
c. Sodium and potassium
d. Calcium and chloride

14. Which of the following statements is correct?
a. Bile is essential for protein metabolism
b. Bile salts function in carbohydrate breakdown
c. Bile is essential for activation of vitamin D
d. Bile is produced in the liver and stored in the gall bladder

15. The talus is a bone in the:
a. Leg
b. Arm
c. Ankle
d. Wrist

16. Kidney stones can be caused by:
a. Hypersecretion of parathormone
b. Hyposecretion of thymosin
c. Hyposecretion of thyroxin
d. None of the above

17. The hormone that regulates the reabsorption of sodium ions into the blood and the secretion of potassium ions into the filtrate is:
a. Parathormone
b. Vasopressin (antidiuretic hormone)
c. Aldosterone
d. Calcitriol

18. The epidermis is:
a. The layer of the skin that provides insulation and storage for fat
b. The layer of the skin that contains blood vessels, nerves, and sweat glands
c. Engaged in a constant process of filtration
d. Engaged in a constant process of cell renewal

19. The brain stem comprises:
a. Right and left cerebral hemispheres
b. Thalamus and hypothalamus
c. Medulla oblongata, pons, and midbrain
d. Cerebellum and cranial nerves

20. Cardiac muscle tissue:
a. Is under voluntary control
b. Is smooth and non-striated
c. Has bundles of branching cells
d. Is found in several hollow organs

21. Which of the following is combined with oxygen in order to produce ATP?
    a. Glycogen
    b. Carbon dioxide
    c. Glucose
    d. ADP

22. The popliteal space can be found:
    a. At the ankles
    b. Behind the knees
    c. Between the ribs
    d. Under the arms

23. Cells that are able to engulf, ingest, and destroy infectious waste and foreign particles are:
    a. Macrophages
    b. Monocytes
    c. Phagocytes
    d. All of the above

24. Which of the following statements is false?
    a. The causes of prostate and testicular cancers are unknown
    b. Polycystic ovary syndrome is cancer of the ovaries
    c. Strong family history is a risk factor for breast cancer
    d. Cervical cancer is often called the "quiet killer"

25. The large intestine is found in:
    a. The upper quadrants of the body
    b. The lower quadrants of the body
    c. All the quadrants of the body
    d. None of the above

26. The pacemaker of the heart can be modified by:
    a. Drugs
    b. The brain
    c. Hormones
    d. All of the above

27. Which of the following statements is correct?
    a. Eccrine glands are larger than apocrine glands
    b. Apocrine glands become active at puberty

    c. Eccrine glands are responsible for body odor
    d. Apocrine glands have a role to play in body temperature

28. Both facial and body massage:
    a. Increase the blood supply to muscle tissue
    b. Relieve muscle fatigue and tension
    c. Hasten the removal of waste products from muscle tissue
    d. All of the above

29. Which of the following is a true statement?
    a. The common name for the epiglottis is the throat
    b. The lungs are contained within the abdominal cavity
    c. The common name for the trachea is the windpipe
    d. The trachea connects the larynx to the bronchioles

30. A ball-and-socket joint is capable of:
    a. Flexion and extension
    b. Adduction and abduction
    c. Rotation and circumduction
    d. All of the above

31. The majority of a cell is made up of:
    a. Organelles
    b. Cytoplasm
    c. Mitochondria
    d. Nucleus

32. Massage should be performed:
    a. Toward the feet
    b. Toward the lymph nodes
    c. Away from the heart
    d. Away from the head

33. The cause of hiatus hernia is:
    a. Hereditary
    b. Trauma
    c. Bacterial
    d. Unknown

34. Amenorrhea can be caused by:
    a. The menopause
    b. Pregnancy
    c. Anorexia nervosa
    d. All of the above

35. The bladder is:
    a. Situated in the pelvic cavity behind the symphysis pubis
    b. Attached to the posterior abdominal wall
    c. Behind the urethra
    d. In the abdominal cavity behind the intestines

36. Which of the following is not true?
    a. Sun exposure accelerates aging of the skin
    b. Smoking, alcohol, and caffeine affect the appearance of the skin
    c. Exposure to the sun causes less melanin to be produced
    d. Exposure to the sun can harm the skin but can also improve certain conditions

37. Which of these is false regarding cerebrovascular accident (stroke)?
    a. Speech is always affected
    b. It is caused by disruption of blood supply to a part of the brain
    c. High blood pressure is a risk factor
    d. There can be sudden weakness on one side of the body

38. Which is the correct composition below for inspired air?
    a. 4.5% carbon dioxide and 16% oxygen
    b. 0.04% carbon dioxide and 21% oxygen
    c. 0.04% carbon dioxide and 16% oxygen
    d. 4.5% carbon dioxide and 21% oxygen

39. Which of the following does not contain yellow elastic tissue?
    a. Bronchial tubes
    b. Lung tissue
    c. Urinary bladder
    d. Aorta

40. Gangrene:
    a. May be a complication of diabetes mellitus
    b. May result from frostbite

c. May result from severe arteriosclerosis

d. All of the above

41. The hormone that is the "opposite" to insulin is:
a. Glucagon
b. Glycogen
c. Glucose
d. Glycolysis

42. The hormone responsible for the maintenance of pregnancy is:
a. Oxytocin
b. Prolactin
c. Progesterone
d. Testosterone

43. "Haustra" are to be found:
a. In the small intestine
b. In the large intestine
c. In the stomach
d. In the liver

44. Nephritis:
a. Can occur anywhere in the kidney
b. Can be known as Bright's disease

c. Is inflammation of the kidneys
d. All of the above

45. Synovial fluid cannot be found:
a. In diarthrotic joints
b. In bursae
c. Within the knee joint
d. In a long bone

46. Which of the following is not a true statement?
a. Joints between the bones of the cranium are fused at birth
b. The "soft spots" found on the cranium are called fontanelles
c. The cranium is composed of eight bones
d. Joints between the bones of the cranium are called sutures

47. An increase in metabolism, fast heart rate, anxiety, and heat intolerance are all symptoms of:
a. Myxedema
b. Seasonal affective disorder
c. Pregnancy
d. Thyrotoxicosis

48. Phagocytosis means:
a. The process by which antibodies are produced
b. The process by which infections are "remembered" and destroyed
c. The process by which foreign particles are engulfed and digested
d. The process by which B and T lymphocytes become mature

49. The cervix lies:
a. In the neck
b. Between the vagina and uterus
c. Between the ovary and fallopian tube
d. In the breast

50. A fever:
a. Is an elevation of core temperature
b. Intensifies the effects of the body's defenses
c. Inhibits the activity of some pathogens
d. All of the above

Practice Quiz 8

1. The fallopian tubes are lined with:
a. Squamous epithelium
b. Ciliated epithelium
c. Cuboid epithelium
d. Transitional epithelium

2. Which part of the tooth acts as a barrier against acids?
a. Enamel
b. Root
c. Crown
d. Neck

3. Which of the following is not true?
a. The size of the vertebrae increases down to the lower back in order to support the weight of the body
b. Although vertebrae differ in size and shape, they all share a similar structural pattern
c. The discs found between the vertebrae form diarthrotic joints in order to facilitate free movement
d. The lumbar vertebrae provide attachment for the large muscles of the back

4. Which of these is not a function of cerebrospinal fluid?
a. Protects the CNS by fighting infection
b. Acts as a shock absorber
c. Acts as a medium for exchange of nutrients and waste
d. Maintains constant pressure around the CNS

5. Which of the following are all functions of the urinary system?
a. Filters waste, regulates blood flow, excretes hormones, maintains pH

b. Filters blood, forms urine, maintains pH, regulates fluid and salt balance
c. Maintains calcium balance, forms feces, regulates fluids, excretes urine
d. Regulates blood flow, filters lymph, assists mineral balance, forms urine

6. **Which of the following best describes the functions of the skin?**
a. Heat regulation, secretion, excretion, sensation
b. Protection, sensation, production of vitamin E, absorption
c. Excretion, protection, heat regulation, circulation
d. Absorption, production of vitamin D, respiration, protection

7. **Which gases are exchanged in the lungs?**
a. Oxygen and nitrogen
b. Oxygen and carbon dioxide
c. Oxygen and carbon monoxide
d. Oxygen and air

8. **Lymphocytes:**
a. Engulf and destroy harmful microbes
b. Produce antigens
c. Selectively filter white cells and platelets
d. Produce antibodies

9. **Which of these hormones are secreted by the posterior pituitary gland?**
a. Melanocyte-stimulating hormone and prolactin
b. Follicle-stimulating hormone and luteinizing hormone
c. Growth hormone and thyroid-stimulating hormone
d. Oxytocin and vasopressin (antidiuretic hormone)

10. **Why is the right kidney slightly lower down than the left?**
a. Because the right kidney is heavier than the left
b. Because the left kidney is pushed upward by the spleen

c. Because the right kidney is pushed down by the liver
d. Because there is less fat covering the right kidney

11. **Which of the following is correct?**
a. A sagittal plane divides the body into unequal portions
b. A frontal plane divides the body into anterior and posterior portions
c. An oblique plane divides the body into equal portions
d. A transverse plane divides the body vertically into right and left portions

12. **The part of the hair that can be seen above the skin surface is the:**
a. Bulb
b. Shaft
c. Follicle
d. Root

13. **Muscle fatigue is not caused by:**
a. A lack of ATP
b. A build-up of lactic acid
c. The inability of the muscle to contract
d. Too much glycogen

14. **An exaggerated lumbar curve characterized by a sway back and lower backache is called:**
a. Scoliosis
b. Osteoporosis
c. Lordosis
d. Kyphosis

15. **A blood vessel made up of a single layer of endothelium is:**
a. An artery
b. A capillary
c. An arteriole
d. A vein

16. **The purpose of the C-shaped cartilage in the trachea is to:**
a. Allow the esophagus to expand
b. Prevent collapse of the trachea
c. Both of these
d. Neither of these

17. **Which of these hormones has an effect upon the skeletal system?**
a. Calcitonin
b. Parathormone
c. Growth hormone
d. All of the above

18. **Muscles that assist, and are found alongside, the prime mover are called:**
a. Synergists
b. Agonists
c. Antagonists
d. All of the above

19. **Hodgkin's disease is:**
a. Cancer of red blood cells
b. Cancer of the tonsils
c. Cancer of the spleen
d. Cancer of lymphocytes

20. **Ovulation usually occurs:**
a. Mid-cycle
b. At the start of the cycle
c. Toward the end of the cycle
d. None of the above

21. **Which organ is essential to life?**
a. The pancreas
b. The stomach
c. The gall bladder
d. All of the above

22. **The function of the heart valves is:**
a. To pump blood at a steady rate
b. To ensure blood flow to the lungs
c. To divide the heart into chambers
d. To prevent backflow of blood

23. **The phrenic nerve is part of the _____ plexus.**
a. Cervical
b. Brachial
c. Lumbar
d. Sacral

24. **Chromosomes are made up of:**
a. ATP
b. DNA
c. RNA
d. CHO

25. The renal pelvis is connected to the:
   a. Ureter
   b. Bladder
   c. Urethra
   d. None of the above

26. Which one of these statements is false regarding angina pectoris?
   a. It is caused by insufficient blood supply to the heart muscle
   b. The pain of angina is not relieved by rest and relaxation
   c. It can be brought on by exercise or emotional stress
   d. The pain may spread from the chest into the arm or jaw

27. Which of the following statements is untrue regarding antigens?
   a. They may activate the immune response
   b. They may trigger an allergic reaction
   c. They can come from transplanted organs such as a heart or kidney
   d. They are usually produced by the body's own cells

28. The adrenal cortex produces _____ groups of hormones.
   a. 2
   b. 3
   c. 7
   d. 9

29. Which of these glands produce oil to protect the skin and hair?
   a. Sebaceous
   b. Sweat
   c. Apocrine
   d. Eccrine

30. Which muscle below does not flex the forearm?
   a. Biceps brachii
   b. Biceps femoris
   c. Brachialis
   d. Brachioradialis

31. The walls of the alveoli are lined with _____ to aid diffusion.
   a. Cuboid epithelium
   b. Ciliated epithelium
   c. Squamous epithelium
   d. Stratified epithelium

32. An "autoimmune" disease is:
   a. An inherited disease
   b. One that a person suffers from and no one else catches it
   c. One where the body's defense system attacks its own tissues
   d. A disease that automatically cures itself after a period of time

33. Which of the following is an incorrect statement regarding the cardiac cycle?
   a. It can be a cause of high blood pressure
   b. It lasts approximately 0.8 seconds
   c. It comprises all the events associated with one heart beat
   d. It comprises both systole and diastole

34. The vulva:
   a. Is part of the vagina
   b. Houses the external genitalia in women
   c. Houses the external genitalia in men
   d. Is part of the scrotal sac

35. The large intestine consists of:
   a. Cecum, colon, rectum, jejunum
   b. Rectum, ascending colon, ileum, descending colon
   c. Colon, duodenum, jejunum, anal canal
   d. Cecum, rectum, anal canal, colon

36. If you stand in the anatomical position with your palms facing forward and turn your palms toward your thighs so that they face backward, you have just:
   a. Abducted your forearms
   b. Adducted your forearms
   c. Laterally rotated your forearms
   d. Medially rotated your forearms

37. The water-soluble vitamins are:
   a. A and B
   b. B and C
   c. D and K
   d. E and C

38. The pelvic cavity does not contain:
   a. The gall bladder
   b. The reproductive organs
   c. The urinary bladder
   d. Part of the large intestine

39. Water and salts are reabsorbed in the:
   a. Glomerulus
   b. Loop of Henle
   c. Efferent arteriole
   d. All of the above

40. Tinea unguium is:
   a. Psoriasis of the nail
   b. Discoloration of the nail caused by viral infection
   c. Ringworm of the nail caused by fungal infection
   d. Bacterial infection of the nail fold

41. Dyspnea is:
   a. Painful or difficult breathing
   b. No breathing
   c. Increased rate of breathing
   d. Very slow breathing

42. The butterfly-shaped endocrine gland wrapped around the trachea is the:
   a. Thymus
   b. Thyroid
   c. Thalamus
   d. Hypothalamus

43. If fertilization occurs, which structure houses a fetus until birth?
    a. Fallopian tubes
    b. Ovaries
    c. Uterus
    d. Urethra

44. Hinge joints are capable of:
    a. Abduction and adduction
    b. Rotation and circumduction
    c. Flexion and extension
    d. None of the above

45. The taste buds are located on the tongue in elevations called _____.
    a. Papillomas
    b. Papillae
    c. Pustules
    d. Pyramids

46. Which of the following is false?
    a. The majority of people who suffer from anorexia nervosa are female
    b. Anorexia nervosa can lead to death
    c. Anorexia nervosa has a high incidence in countries where there is food shortage
    d. Amenorrhea accompanies anorexia nervosa

47. A clouding over of the lens of the eye commonly found in older people is:
    a. A corneal ulcer
    b. A cataract
    c. A glaucoma
    d. Conjunctivitis

48. Which of the following best describes the characteristics of muscle tissue?
    a. Excitability, conductivity, enforceability, irritability
    b. Elasticity, extensibility, excitability, contractility
    c. Contractility, sensitivity, conductivity, extensibility
    d. Irritability, excitability, extensibility, enforceability

49. Which of the following is a by-product of cellular respiration?
    a. Glucose
    b. Lactic acid
    c. Carbon dioxide
    d. Oxygen

50. The correct order in the conduction system through the heart is:
    a. Atrioventricular node, bundle of His, sinoatrial node, Purkinje fibers
    b. Sinoatrial node, atrioventricular node, bundle of His, Purkinje fibers
    c. Sinoatrial node, Purkinje fibers, bundle of His, atrioventricular node
    d. Purkinje fibers, atrioventricular node, bundle of His, sinoatrial node

Practice Quiz 9

1. Efferent neurons conduct impulses:
    a. From CNS to muscles and glands
    b. From muscles and glands to CNS
    c. From PNS to CNS
    d. From sensory receptors to PNS

2. The phalanges are examples of:
    a. Short bones
    b. Long bones
    c. Flat bones
    d. Irregular bones

3. The urinary bladder has _____ muscle in its walls.
    a. Voluntary
    b. Cardiac
    c. Smooth
    d. Striated

4. Peyer's patches are found:
    a. In the small intestine
    b. In the spleen
    c. In the large intestine
    d. In the liver

5. The perineum is located:
    a. Between the toes
    b. Under the arms
    c. Behind the knees
    d. Between the legs

6. An average normal pregnancy lasts _____ weeks.
    a. 20
    b. 30
    c. 40
    d. 50

7. Gases carried in the blood are:
    a. Oxygen
    b. Nitrogen
    c. Carbon dioxide
    d. All of the above

8. Which of these structures is not found within the conducting zone?
    a. Alveolus
    b. Bronchus

c. Nose
d. Pharynx

9. The link between the endocrine and nervous systems is considered to be the:
   a. Midbrain
   b. Medulla oblongata
   c. Hypothalamus
   d. Thalamus

10. The surface area of food to be digested is increased by the work of the:
    a. Tongue
    b. Teeth
    c. Saliva
    d. Uvula

11. Which of the statements below is true of fascia?
    a. It is made of dense, irregular connective tissue
    b. It supports the nerves and blood vessels that support the muscles
    c. It separates muscles into different groups
    d. All are true

12. The correct term for shedding of skin cells is:
    a. Detoxification
    b. Desquamation
    c. Exfoliation
    d. Excretion

13. It is possible for the body to survive without the:
    a. Liver
    b. Red bone marrow
    c. Spleen
    d. None of the above

14. Which of these statements is true?
    a. Reproduction is possible before puberty
    b. Reproduction is possible after the menopause
    c. It is not possible for men to reproduce after the age of 55
    d. It is possible to reproduce after the menarche

15. Prolactin targets the:
    a. Uterus to contract
    b. Development of secondary sex characteristics
    c. Body clock
    d. Mammary glands to produce milk

16. Looking at a picture of the heart, what is the bottom left-hand chamber called?
    a. Right atrium
    b. Right ventricle
    c. Left atrium
    d. Left ventricle

17. Thickening and scarring of the lung tissue is known as:
    a. Pulmonary fibrosis
    b. Sarcoidosis
    c. Sinusitis
    d. Pulmonary embolism

18. The semimembranosus is part of the _____.
    a. Adductors
    b. Quadriceps
    c. Hamstrings
    d. None of the above

19. The root, shaft, and follicle are all parts of which structure of the integumentary system?
    a. Nail
    b. Hair
    c. Skin
    d. All of the above

20. Hearing a constant buzzing or other noise that other people cannot hear could be:
    a. Vertigo
    b. Otitis media
    c. Tinnitus
    d. Earache

21. The atlas and axis form what sort of joint?
    a. Hinge
    b. Pivot
    c. Ball-and-socket
    d. Condyloid

22. A body system not involved in excretion is:
    a. The integumentary system
    b. The nervous system
    c. The respiratory system
    d. The urinary system

23. Which of the following vitamins is water soluble and not fat soluble?
    a. Vitamin C
    b. Vitamin D
    c. Vitamin E
    d. Vitamin K

24. The structures that increase surface area in the digestive system are the:
    a. Villi
    b. Plicae circulares
    c. Microvilli
    d. All of the above

25. Amenorrhea occurs:
    a. In pregnancy
    b. Before puberty
    c. During the menopause
    d. All of the above

26. Deoxygenated blood is transported back to the heart by the:
    a. Aorta
    b. Venae cavae
    c. Coronary veins
    d. Pulmonary veins

27. Lateral epicondylitis is:
    a. Housemaid's knee
    b. Golfer's elbow
    c. Tennis elbow
    d. None of the above

28. Pes planus affects:
    a. Cervical spine
    b. Arches of the feet
    c. Cartilage in the knee
    d. All the joints in the body

29. Which of the following statements is correct?
    a. More lymphatic vessels enter a lymph node than leave it
    b. The majority of lymph is collected by the right lymphatic duct

c. Creamy-colored lymph drains into the cisterna chyli from the spleen
d. All the above

30. The seminiferous tubules, sustentacular cells, and Leydig cells are all to be found in:
a. The ovaries
b. The testes
c. The breast
d. The placenta

31. Which of the following conditions can children be vaccinated against?
a. Whooping cough
b. Asthma
c. Asbestosis
d. Sinusitis

32. The correct order of structures in the digestive system through which food passes is:
a. Mouth, stomach, liver, large intestine, rectum
b. Esophagus, stomach, duodenum, pancreas, colon
c. Mouth, esophagus, stomach, small intestine, large intestine
d. Esophagus, ileum, pancreas, cecum, rectum

33. Which of the following statements is incorrect?
a. The internal urethral sphincter is composed of smooth muscle fibers
b. Emptying or voiding the bladder is known as micturition
c. The walls of the bladder contain stretch receptors
d. The internal urethral sphincter is under voluntary control

34. Which statement is true regarding sickle cell anemia?
a. The hemoglobin of sufferers bends the red blood cells into a crescent shape
b. People who suffer from it have a high resistance to malaria
c. It is a genetic disorder
d. All of the above

35. Which of the muscles below lies deepest in the body?
a. Transversus abdominis
b. Rectus abdominis
c. External obliques
d. Internal obliques

36. Bacterial infection of the skin surrounding the nails is called:
a. Leuconychia
b. Anonychia
c. Paronychia
d. Koilonychia

37. Gigantism does not occur after puberty is complete because:
a. Children have smaller pituitary glands
b. The long bones of an adult have stopped lengthening
c. The growth hormone is no longer secreted after puberty
d. All of the above

38. Stimulation of the sympathetic nervous system would result in:
a. Increased heart rate, increase in gastric juice, bronchodilation
b. Increased heart rate, reduced peristalsis, dilated pupils
c. Bronchodilation, constricted pupils, increased saliva
d. Decreased saliva, bronchoconstriction, dilated pupils

39. Oxygen and carbon dioxide pass through the cell membrane by:
a. Simple diffusion
b. Vesicular transport
c. Facilitated diffusion
d. Active transport

40. Polycystic ovary syndrome may cause:
a. Weight gain
b. Chest and facial hair
c. Infertility
d. All of the above

41. Which statement is true of neurotransmitters?
a. They are always excitatory
b. They are always inhibitory
c. They can also be a hormone
d. They are stored in the synaptic cleft

42. Bursae are found:
a. Between tendons and bones
b. Between ligaments and bones
c. Between muscles and bones
d. All of the above

43. The renal tubule has a/an _____ lining.
a. Epithelial
b. Mucous membrane
c. Serous membrane
d. Muscular

44. Anaphylactic shock is:
a. A disease-causing microorganism
b. An extremely severe allergic reaction
c. A butterfly rash across the nose and cheeks
d. An extremely painful sore throat

45. Cytokinesis is:
a. The process whereby cells are able to move
b. The process during which cells die
c. The process by which the cytoplasm divides
d. All of the above

46. Which protein molecule in red blood cells has an enormous affinity for oxygen?
a. Prothrombin
b. Globulin
c. Albumin
d. Hemoglobin

47. Which one of the following is a false statement?
a. Jaundice is a symptom, not a sign of disease
b. Jaundice causes yellowing of the skin
c. Jaundice can occur temporarily in newborns
d. Jaundice is caused by high levels of bilirubin

48. Which of the statements below is not true of psoriasis?
a. It is improved by exposure to the sun
b. It shows raised red patches with silvery scales

c. It may run in families
d. It is a viral skin condition

49. **Which is the correct order of lymph flow within the lymphatic system?**
    a. Capillaries, ducts, subclavian veins, vessels

b. Capillaries, vessels, ducts, subclavian veins
c. Subclavian veins, ducts, vessels, capillaries
d. Vessels, subclavian veins, capillaries, ducts

50. _____ result from protein breakdown.
    a. Fatty acids
    b. Glucose
    c. Amino acids
    d. Glycogen

Practice Quiz 10

1. **Which of the following is a false statement regarding muscle tone?**
   a. It is absent during sleep or unconsciousness
   b. It maintains posture
   c. It is improved by exercise and massage
   d. It is when every muscle fiber is relaxed

2. **Of the cells in the blood, 99% of them are:**
   a. White cells
   b. Red cells
   c. Platelets
   d. Antibodies

3. **What is the function of transitional epithelial tissue?**
   a. To protect underlying organs
   b. To move substances along a passageway
   c. To line organs that secrete substances
   d. To allow organs to distend or expand

4. **Difficulty in childbirth, lifting heavy objects, chronic coughing, or constipation could result in:**
   a. Vaginitis
   b. Toxic shock syndrome
   c. Prolapse of the uterus
   d. Prostatitis

5. **The structure that drains lymph from the right shoulder is the:**
   a. Tonsils
   b. Right lymphatic duct
   c. Thoracic duct
   d. Right subclavian vein

6. **Which of the following is a false statement?**
   a. The kidneys help in the production of white blood cells
   b. The kidneys play a very important part in homeostasis
   c. The kidneys help to regulate blood pressure
   d. The kidneys help the body to use vitamin D

7. **Exchange of gases takes place in the _____ zone.**
   a. Ventilatory
   b. Conducting
   c. Respiratory
   d. All of the above

8. **The "master gland" of the body is the:**
   a. Pancreas
   b. Pituitary
   c. Pineal
   d. Parathyroid

9. **The skin protects the body by:**
   a. Forming a physical barrier against microorganisms
   b. Tanning in response to exposure to ultraviolet radiation
   c. Exhibiting erythema and/or rashes in response to antigens
   d. All of the above

10. **Which of the following is a false statement regarding deglutition?**
    a. It interrupts breathing
    b. It is a mechanical process

c. It takes approximately two seconds
d. It is involuntary

11. **The brain, meninges, and spinal cord are part of the:**
    a. Central nervous system
    b. Peripheral nervous system
    c. Sympathetic nervous system
    d. Parasympathetic nervous system

12. **An exaggerated thoracic curve, common in the elderly and which can be a result of osteoporosis, is:**
    a. Scoliosis
    b. Kyphosis
    c. Lordosis
    d. Spondylosis

13. **Luteinizing hormone:**
    a. Stimulates ovulation
    b. Stimulates production of testosterone
    c. Stimulates production of estrogen
    d. All of the above

14. **In general, disorders of the muscular system are accompanied by:**
    a. Pain
    b. Limitation of movement
    c. Inflammation
    d. All of the above

15. **Which of the following is not a protein?**
    a. Steroid
    b. Enzyme
    c. Antibody
    d. Hormone

16. Poor sperm motility may cause:
    a. Impotence
    b. Menorrhagia
    c. Infertility
    d. Prostatitis

17. Which of the following is a false statement regarding the spleen?
    a. It destroys old and worn out erythrocytes
    b. It filters lymph and blood
    c. It produces lymphocytes
    d. It stores platelets and blood

18. "Goosebumps" are:
    a. An attempt to lower body temperature
    b. Caused by contraction of the arrector pili muscle
    c. A bacterial infection of hair follicles
    d. Caused by blocked sebaceous glands

19. The pectoral girdle consists of:
    a. Ribs and vertebrae
    b. Radius and ulna
    c. Clavicle and scapula
    d. Sacrum and pubis

20. The nasal cavity is lined with a _____ membrane.
    a. Mucous
    b. Serous
    c. Synovial
    d. Glandular

21. Parkinson's disease is characterized by:
    a. Chronic infection
    b. Involuntary muscle tremors and rigidity
    c. Recurrent seizures
    d. Insomnia

22. Which of the following conditions is not a type of repetitive strain injury?
    a. Shin splints
    b. Housemaid's knee
    c. Fibromyalgia
    d. Tendonitis

23. Which artery supplies the heart muscle itself with blood?
    a. Coronary
    b. Carotid
    c. Cardiac
    d. Cephalic

24. Blood and lymphatic vessels, nerves, and the ureters enter and leave the kidney at the:
    a. Pelvis
    b. Hilum
    c. Cortex
    d. Medulla

25. Androgens are not responsible for:
    a. Secondary sex characteristics in women
    b. Growth of pubic and axillary hair in both sexes
    c. The lowering of the voice
    d. Secondary sex characteristics in men

26. What sort of infection is athlete's foot?
    a. Bacterial
    b. Fungal
    c. Viral
    d. None of the above

27. The vast majority of absorption takes place in the:
    a. Stomach
    b. Colon
    c. Small intestine
    d. Liver

28. Which of the following is an incorrect statement?
    a. Simple cuboidal epithelium covers the surface of the ovaries
    b. Adipose tissue is found in the mammary glands
    c. Smooth muscle tissue is found in the myometrium
    d. Ciliated epithelial tissue lines the vagina

29. The presence of air in the pleural space is called:
    a. Pleurisy
    b. Pneumothorax
    c. Pneumonia
    d. None of the above

30. Which of the following muscles is named by its origin and insertion?
    a. Levator palpebrae superioris
    b. Deltoid
    c. Sternocleidomastoid
    d. Corrugator supercilii

31. DNA is the _____ of the cell.
    a. Genetic material
    b. Detoxification area
    c. Control center
    d. Recycling center

32. Onycholysis is:
    a. Nail biting
    b. Overgrowth of the cuticle
    c. Separation of the nail from its bed
    d. Ingrowing toenail

33. Which statement is false?
    a. The muscular layer of the stomach is called rugae
    b. The stomach can stretch and hold up to four 1 gallon (4 liters)
    c. The inner mucosal layer of the stomach contains gastric glands
    d. Some of the muscle fibers in the stomach are arranged obliquely

34. Which is true of the autonomic nervous system?
    a. It is under the control of the will
    b. It is an involuntary system
    c. It is part of the CNS
    d. It is controlled by the cerebellum

35. Which bone is butterfly-shaped and lies at the base of the skull?
    a. Temporal
    b. Occipital
    c. Sphenoid
    d. Ethmoid

36. The cardiovascular system regulates temperature by:
    a. Oxygenation and deoxygenation of the blood
    b. Contraction and relaxation of the heart

c. Vasoconstriction and vasodilation of blood vessels
d. All of the above

37. Macrophages:
   a. Are also phagocytes
   b. Can be "wandering" or "fixed"
   c. Develop from monocytes
   d. All of the above

38. Insulin cannot be given orally into the stomach because:
   a. The amount needed would cause the tablets to be too large
   b. The enzymes needed are found only in the skin
   c. It is a protein hormone and would be digested by enzymes there
   d. None of the above

39. A high-fat, low-fiber diet may predispose one to:
   a. Gallstones
   b. Cancer of the colon
   c. Appendicitis
   d. All of the above

40. An average heart rate is between:
   a. 40 and 60 beats per minute
   b. 50 and 70 beats per minute
   c. 60 and 80 beats per minute
   d. 80 and 100 beats per minute

41. The four most abundant elements, which make up about 96%, of the body are:
   a. Carbon, oxygen, phosphorus, calcium
   b. Oxygen, nitrogen, sodium, carbon
   c. Carbon, oxygen, nitrogen, hydrogen
   d. Hydrogen, calcium, phosphorus, sodium

42. The process of oogenesis is:
   a. Production of male gametes
   b. Production of female gametes
   c. Production of male gonads
   d. Production of female gonads

43. The renal tubule includes the:
   a. Loop of Henle
   b. Distal convoluted tubule
   c. Proximal convoluted tubule
   d. All of the above

44. Yellow elastic tissue can be found in:
   a. Lung tissue
   b. Bronchial tubes
   c. Trachea
   d. All of the above

45. Which of the following cranial nerves is purely a sensory nerve?
   a. Optic (II)
   b. Facial (VII)
   c. Vagus (X)
   d. Hypoglossal (XII)

46. Ball-and-socket joints are found:
   a. At the knee and elbow only
   b. At the shoulder and hip only
   c. At the wrist and foot only
   d. None of the above

47. Centrioles are:
   a. Rod-like organelles that play an important part in mitosis
   b. Networks of fluid-filled cisterns for chemical reactions and transportation
   c. Vesicles containing digestive enzymes to break down and destroy foreign substances
   d. Chromosomes massed together, which separate during cell division

48. Mechanical digestion includes:
   a. Peristalsis
   b. Segmentation
   c. Stomach churning
   d. All of the above

49. A client who reports a painless enlargement of lymph nodes under her arm should:
   a. Do more exercise as the lymphatic system may be blocked
   b. Book some massage sessions
   c. Consult her doctor immediately
   d. Change her diet

50. Enuresis is common in:
   a. Childhood
   b. Teenagers
   c. Middle age
   d. Old age

Practice Quiz 11

1. Hormones are produced by endocrine glands in response to:
   a. Hormonal stimulation
   b. Chemical changes in the blood
   c. Neural stimulation
   d. All of the above

2. The mammary artery can be found in the region of the:
   a. Breast
   b. Back
   c. Abdomen
   d. Heart

3. Which of the following is a true statement?
   a. White blood cells are larger than red ones but there are fewer of them
   b. Red blood cells carry oxygen and have a vital role in defense
   c. White blood cells contain hemoglobin, which gives them their pale color
   d. There are several different types of red blood cell but only one type of white blood cell

4. Apocrine glands excrete:
   a. Watery sweat
   b. Oil
   c. Fatty or milky sweat
   d. Serous fluid

5. Which part of the urinary system transports urine from the kidneys to the bladder?
   a. Pelvis
   b. Ureter
   c. Cortex
   d. Urethra

6. There are _____ bones in the axial skeleton and _____ in the appendicular skeleton.
   a. 60 and 206
   b. 80 and 126
   c. 126 and 80
   d. 206 and 60

7. Which of the following statements is true?
   a. Enzymes either speed up or slow down the rate of chemical reactions
   b. Enzymes are not affected by the acidic environment of the gut
   c. The digestion of food relies on the presence of enzymes
   d. All of the above

8. In the male reproductive system, sperm mature in the:
   a. Penis
   b. Epididymis
   c. Prostate gland
   d. Vas deferens

9. Mucosa-associated lymphoid tissue (MALT) is found in the:
   a. Gastrointestinal tract
   b. Respiratory airways
   c. Urinary tract
   d. All of the above

10. The kidneys are not affected by:
    a. Diabetes mellitus
    b. Diabetes insipidus
    c. Addison's disease
    d. Graves' disease

11. A person suffering from a severe infection would have _____ in their blood.
    a. An increased number of red cells
    b. A decreased number of white cells
    c. An increased number of white cells

    d. A decreased number of platelets

12. The virus that causes chickenpox can reactivate in later life as:
    a. Rubella
    b. Herpes zoster
    c. Herpes simplex
    d. Rubeola

13. The study of the nervous system is:
    a. Histology
    b. Nephrology
    c. Craniopathy
    d. Neurology

14. The outermost layer of connective tissue that encircles the whole muscle is the:
    a. Endomysium
    b. Epimysium
    c. Perimysium
    d. Deep fascia

15. The main central shaft of a long bone is the:
    a. Diaphysis
    b. Epiphysis
    c. Endosteum
    d. Periosteum

16. The function of the large intestine is:
    a. Absorption of water
    b. Defecation
    c. Absorption of vitamin K
    d. All of the above

17. The function of the nose is to _____ the incoming air.
    a. Moisten
    b. Warm
    c. Filter
    d. All of the above

18. Popliteal nodes are located:
    a. In the abdomen
    b. In front of the elbow
    c. Behind the knee
    d. In the neck

19. Which of the following is a false statement?
    a. Progesterone is only produced in the second half of the menstrual cycle
    b. The menstrual flow occurs as levels of estrogen and progesterone decline
    c. The secretory phase occurs just before the menstrual period
    d. The corpus luteum is produced under the influence of FSH

20. The islets of Langerhans are found:
    a. In the scrotum
    b. In the pancreas
    c. Either side of the thyroid
    d. Above the pituitary

21. Organic substances are ones that contain:
    a. Carbon
    b. Oxygen
    c. Nitrogen
    d. Hydrogen

22. The neurotransmitter that is released at the neuromuscular junction and triggers a muscle action potential is:
    a. Norepinephrine (noradrenaline)
    b. Dopamine
    c. Acetylcholine
    d. Epinephrine (adrenaline)

23. In the nephron, the afferent arteriole divides into the:
    a. Glomerulus
    b. Efferent arteriole
    c. Collecting duct
    d. Bowman's capsule

24. The brain is responsible for:
    a. Controlling reflex actions
    b. Conducting impulses from sensory receptors
    c. Making and storing memories
    d. None of the above

25. Which of the following may be caused by cigarette smoking?
    a. Bronchitis
    b. Emphysema

c. Lung cancer
d. All of the above

26. Lymph nodes are enclosed in:
    a. Dense connective tissue
    b. Smooth muscle tissue
    c. Transitional epithelium
    d. Neuroglial tissue

27. The left atrium receives
    _____ blood from the
    _____.

    a. Oxygenated, lungs
    b. Deoxygenated, body
    c. Oxygenated, right atrium
    d. Deoxygenated, right
       ventricle

28. Facial massage would be
    contraindicated in the presence
    of:
    a. Ephelides
    b. Lentigines
    c. Herpes simplex
    d. Albinism

29. Which of the following
    substances remains in the renal
    tubule?
    a. Amino acids
    b. Uric acid
    c. Glucose
    d. All of the above

30. An enlarged prostate gland:
    a. Causes difficulty in passing
       urine
    b. Can progress to being
       cancerous
    c. Can cause more frequent
       urination
    d. All of the above

31. The mineral content of the blood
    is affected by:
    a. Estrogen
    b. Aldosterone
    c. Testosterone
    d. All of the above

32. The body is always striving
    to maintain a stable internal
    environment by the process of:
    a. Hemostasis
    b. Hemolysis
    c. Homeostasis
    d. Hemopoiesis

33. If the Achilles tendon ruptures/
    tears, what action will not be
    possible?
    a. Waving
    b. Walking
    c. Breathing
    d. Eating

34. In this fracture the broken ends
    of the bone pierce the skin and
    infection may enter the wound:
    a. Compound
    b. Simple
    c. Comminuted
    d. Greenstick

35. The "intrinsic factor" is necessary
    for the absorption of vitamin
    _____ from the ileum.
    a. B1
    b. D
    c. K
    d. B12

36. Spina bifida:
    a. Is a condition of old age
    b. Is present at birth
    c. Develops at puberty
    d. Is triggered by the
       menopause

37. For normal expiration to take
    place:
    a. Atmospheric pressure must
       be greater than the pressure
       in the lungs
    b. The pressure in the lungs
       must be greater than
       atmospheric pressure
    c. The pressure must be equal
       in both areas
    d. The pressure varies
       depending on the amount of
       activity being done

38. Calcium, potassium, iron, and
    chlorine are all examples of:
    a. Fatty acids
    b. Vitamins
    c. Monosaccharides
    d. Minerals

39. The largest organ of the body
    is the:
    a. Liver
    b. Heart
    c. Skin
    d. Brain

40. Which of the following
    conditions is the result of a
    clotting disorder?
    a. Myocardial infarction
    b. Hemophilia
    c. Epistaxis
    d. Pernicious anemia

41. Congenital absence of a nail is
    called:
    a. Anonychia
    b. Paronychia
    c. Leuconychia
    d. Koilonychia

42. Which of the following muscles
    moves the thumb?
    a. Flexor carpi ulnaris
    b. Flexor digitorum
       superficialis
    c. Flexor carpi radialis
    d. Flexor pollicis brevis

43. Stones found in the urinary
    system are called renal
    _____.
    a. Cysts
    b. Calculi
    c. Calyces
    d. Cusps

44. In relation to the vertebral
    column the cervical curve
    develops when:
    a. A baby is able to walk
    b. A baby is able to stand up
    c. A baby is able to sit up
    d. A baby is able to hold its
       head up

45. Which of the following is true?
    a. Digestion occurs at the
       brush border
    b. Digested proteins enter the
       bloodstream via the lacteals
    c. Crypts of Lieberkühn are
       situated in the duodenum
    d. Brunner's glands are situated
       in the stomach

46. Dysmenorrhea means:
    a. Painful menstruation
    b. Infertility
    c. Lack of menstruation
    d. Inflammation in the pelvis

47. The cauda equina is part of the:
   a. Autonomic nervous system
   b. Brain
   c. Spinal cord
   d. Meninges

48. Oxygen is transported in the blood by:
   a. Plasma
   b. Red blood cells
   c. Platelets
   d. White blood cells

49. Which condition affects the normal development of leucocytes and is known to invade organs, such as the liver and spleen, causing infection, bleeding, and anemia?
   a. Lymphoma
   b. AIDS
   c. SLE
   d. Leukemia

50. Which of the following is a false statement?
   a. The amount of urine passed daily is always the same
   b. The amount of urine passed daily is affected by how much exercise we do
   c. The amount of urine passed daily is affected by our general state of health
   d. The amount of urine passed daily is affected by hormones

Practice Quiz 12

1. The name of the membrane that encloses the lungs is the:
   a. Pharynx
   b. Pericardium
   c. Peritoneum
   d. Pleura

2. Breaking down large droplets of fat into smaller ones is known as:
   a. Deamination
   b. Mastication
   c. Emulsification
   d. Segmentation

3. Which of the following is/are not found in the dermis?
   a. Cells producing melanin
   b. Blood supply
   c. Cells producing histamine
   d. Sweat glands

4. When does the thymus gland begin to atrophy?
   a. After puberty
   b. Before puberty
   c. During childhood
   d. During the menopause

5. A girl of 14 is much smaller than her peer group and has average-sized parents. She could be lacking in _____ (hormone).
   a. ACTH
   b. hGH
   c. LH
   d. ADH (vasopressin)

6. Which of the following substances should not normally be present in urine?
   a. Water
   b. Glucose
   c. Urea
   d. Uric acid

7. The process of stopping bleeding is called:
   a. Homeopathy
   b. Homeostasis
   c. Hemostasis
   d. Hemopoiesis

8. Which myofilament gives skeletal muscle its dark banding?
   a. Titin
   b. Myosin
   c. Actin
   d. Troponin

9. The hormone that is responsible for the onset of labor is:
   a. Hormone replacement therapy
   b. Prolactin
   c. Luteinizing hormone
   d. Oxytocin

10. The study of body tissues is called:
   a. Anatomy
   b. Histology
   c. Cytology
   d. Physiology

11. Efferent neurons conduct impulses:
   a. From CNS to muscles and glands
   b. From muscles and glands to CNS
   c. From PNS to CNS
   d. From sensory receptors to PNS

12. Which of the following is an incorrect statement?
   a. Mechanical stress is beneficial to the skeletal system
   b. Being bedridden causes bones to become weaker
   c. Aging causes loss of calcium from the bones
   d. Exercise makes the bones more likely to fracture

13. Which of the following statements is false regarding the respiratory system?
   a. The pharynx serves as both an air and a food passageway
   b. The pharynx provides a passageway between the larynx and the bronchi
   c. The larynx contains the vocal cords
   d. The larynx is made of hyaline cartilage

14. The enzymes that digest proteins are known as:
    a. Peptides
    b. Amino acids
    c. Proteases
    d. Substrates

15. The flow of lymph is helped by:
    a. Exercise
    b. Massage
    c. Pressure from skeletal muscles
    d. All of the above

16. The right ventricle sends blood to the:
    a. Lungs
    b. Left ventricle
    c. Right atrium
    d. Body

17. Muscle fibers with a high resistance to fatigue, loaded with mitochondria, and rich in myoglobin will not be of great use to a:
    a. 100-meter runner
    b. Marathon runner
    c. Long-distance swimmer
    d. Long-distance cyclist

18. The correct term for the shoulder blade is the:
    a. Sternum
    b. Scapula
    c. Sesamoid
    d. Sacrum

19. Hyposecretion of the antidiuretic hormone (vasopressin) causes:
    a. Addison's disease
    b. Cushing's syndrome
    c. Diabetes insipidus
    d. Diabetes mellitus

20. Synaptic vesicles contain:
    a. Myelin
    b. Neurotransmitters
    c. Schwann cells
    d. Neurilemma

21. Androgens are produced by:
    a. Testes, ovaries, placenta
    b. Ovaries, adrenal glands in women and men

    c. Adrenal glands in men and women, testes
    d. Testes, placenta, adrenal glands in women only

22. The axillary lymph nodes are situated in the:
    a. Armpits
    b. Groin
    c. Abdomen
    d. Neck

23. Which of the following can be caused by infection and inflammation of the alveoli and surrounding tissues?
    a. Pleurisy
    b. Pneumonia
    c. Hay fever
    d. SARS

24. The function of hydrochloric acid is:
    a. To activate pepsin
    b. An antibacterial
    c. To inhibit salivary amylase
    d. All of the above

25. What happens to the hair during telogen?
    a. Growing
    b. Shedding
    c. Changing
    d. Dividing

26. The afferent arteriole bringing blood to the glomerulus is wider than the efferent arteriole because:
    a. It is nearer to the renal artery
    b. It causes high pressure within the glomerulus
    c. It is carrying many substances to be filtered
    d. It causes the large plasma proteins to be filtered out of the blood

27. The insertion part of a muscle is usually:
    a. Attached to the bone that moves
    b. The fixed point
    c. The origin of the muscle
    d. Attached to the stationary bone

28. The way in which bone tissue is continually replaced throughout life is called:
    a. Retraction
    b. Replacement
    c. Reincarnation
    d. Remodeling

29. Which of the following is true?
    a. Exercise increases the rate and depth of breathing because more carbon dioxide is produced
    b. Exercise increases the rate and depth of breathing because the brain sends messages to the diaphragm to increase its activity
    c. Exercise increases the rate and depth of breathing because there are receptors that monitor the amount of oxygen and carbon dioxide in the blood
    d. All of the above

30. Myxedema is not caused by:
    a. Hypothyroidism
    b. Surgical removal of too much thyroid tissue
    c. Hyperthyroidism
    d. Too little thyroxine

31. We can combat the effect of free radicals by consuming more foods containing:
    a. Fats
    b. Water
    c. Antibiotics
    d. Antioxidants

32. Which of the following statements regarding the liver is false?
    a. It is made up of three lobes arranged in lobules
    b. It is made up of hepatocytes
    c. It contains spaces called sinusoids
    d. It contains phagocytes

33. A viral infection that lowers immunity and increases susceptibility to infections is:
    a. Systemic lupus erythematosus
    b. Infectious mononucleosis

    c. Human immunodeficiency
       virus
    d. Viral encephalitis

34. **Which of the following blood vessels carries oxygenated blood?**
    a. Pulmonary artery
    b. Pulmonary vein
    c. Coronary sinus
    d. None of the above

35. **Which of these statements is incorrect regarding the male urethra?**
    a. It is the terminal duct of the male urinary system
    b. It transports semen and urine out of the body
    c. It is the terminal duct of the male reproductive system
    d. It is a 1½-inch (4 cm) long tube lying behind the symphysis pubis

36. **Bell's palsy is weakness or paralysis of the _____.**
    a. Arms
    b. Legs
    c. Face
    d. Bladder

37. **The cause of rheumatoid arthritis is thought to be:**
    a. Injury
    b. Autoimmune
    c. Bacterial
    d. Age

38. **The dermal papillae:**
    a. Increase the surface area of the papillary layer
    b. Are responsible for fingerprints
    c. Contain capillary networks
    d. All of the above

39. **The odd one out below is:**
    a. Lunula
    b. Acid mantle
    c. Matrix
    d. Cuticle

40. **An autoimmune disease characterized by weakness of skeletal muscles, especially drooping eyelids, could be:**
    a. Myasthenia gravis
    b. Muscular rheumatism
    c. Fibrositis
    d. Metastasis

41. **Which of the following is the correct term for "water-loving"?**
    a. Hydrophobic
    b. Carbohydrate
    c. Hydrophilic
    d. Dehydration

42. **White spots or streaks on nails are called:**
    a. Paronychia
    b. Anonychia
    c. Leuconychia
    d. Koilonychia

43. **Antibodies being passed on in breast milk from mother to baby is an example of:**
    a. Naturally acquired passive immunity
    b. Artificially acquired active immunity
    c. Naturally acquired active immunity
    d. Artificially acquired passive immunity

44. **Epinephrine and norepinephrine are released by the:**
    a. Midbrain
    b. Adrenal cortex
    c. Medulla oblongata
    d. Adrenal medulla

45. **Which of the following statements regarding osmoreceptors is false?**
    a. They detect a decreased level of water in the blood
    b. They detect an increased amount of solutes in the blood
    c. They are situated in the hypothalamus in the brain
    d. They are situated in the medulla oblongata in the brain

46. **Which is a false statement regarding the sense of smell?**
    a. It is interpreted in the brain by the facial nerve
    b. It is closely linked with the sense of taste
    c. It can be affected by a frontal head injury
    d. It is closely linked to emotions and memories

47. **The saphenous veins are to be found in the:**
    a. Trunk
    b. Arms
    c. Legs
    d. Head

48. **Inability to conceive may be caused by:**
    a. Repeated infections of the fallopian tubes
    b. Impotence
    c. Endometriosis
    d. All of the above

49. **Which of the following is a false statement?**
    a. Uremia causes drowsiness, lethargy, and nausea
    b. Uremia is the presence of blood in the urine
    c. Uremia can be fatal if left untreated
    d. Uremia can be caused by renal failure

50. **Cardiac muscle cells are described as being "myogenic." This means:**
    a. They have a constant rhythm
    b. The impulse to beat comes from the endocrine system
    c. They can contract independently of the nervous system
    d. Each cell contracts independently at different times

Practice Quiz 13

1. The liver does not:
   a. Store vitamin C
   b. Store iron and copper
   c. Convert substances into glucose
   d. Convert ammonia into urea

2. Breathing cannot be controlled during:
   a. Singing
   b. Sleeping
   c. Swimming
   d. Shouting

3. During muscle contraction the:
   a. Sarcomeres lengthen
   b. Myofilaments shorten
   c. Sarcomeres shorten
   d. Myofilaments lengthen

4. Killer cells:
   a. Kill tumor cells in the body
   b. Kill the body's own contaminated cells
   c. Kill invading cells
   d. All of the above

5. The testes lie outside the body because:
   a. The internal secretions of the body are too acidic
   b. They are under the influence of the Y chromosome
   c. Sperm survive better at lower temperatures
   d. All of the above

6. Impulses or messages are conducted _____ within the nervous system.
   a. Electrically only
   b. Chemically only
   c. Both electrically and chemically
   d. Neither electrically nor chemically

7. Blood pressure is not affected by the actions of:
   a. Renin
   b. Vasopressin (antidiuretic hormone)
   c. Sodium
   d. Calcitriol

8. Carbohydrates do not contain:
   a. Carbon
   b. Oxygen
   c. Nitrogen
   d. Hydrogen

9. Yellow bone marrow is found in the:
   a. Epiphysis
   b. Diaphysis
   c. Periosteum
   d. None of the above

10. Which of these is a false statement?
    a. Women do not produce androgens
    b. Cortisol helps to deal with long-term stress
    c. Men do not produce progesterone
    d. Epinephrine is known as the "fight-or-flight" hormone

11. Which of the following statements is false?
    a. The heart valves are composed of connective tissue covered by endocardium
    b. The atrioventricular valve on the left has two cusps but the one on the right has three
    c. The atrioventricular valves are called the aortic and pulmonary valves
    d. The semilunar valves lie between the ventricles and the two main arteries leaving the heart

12. Adipocytes are found in the:
    a. Reticular dermis
    b. Subcutaneous layer
    c. Papillary dermis
    d. Epidermis

13. The pyloric sphincter lies between the:
    a. Esophagus and the stomach
    b. Rectum and the anus
    c. Stomach and the duodenum
    d. Bile duct and the duodenum

14. Most muscle fibers in the body are:
    a. Type I (slow oxidative)
    b. Type II (fast oxidative)
    c. Type II (fast glycolytic)
    d. A mixture of all types

15. The function of relaxin is to:
    a. Increase flexibility of the ligaments and joints during labor
    b. Control the menstrual cycle
    c. Control the process of spermatogenesis
    d. Decrease the risk of premature labor

16. Which is a false statement regarding the blood-brain barrier?
    a. Its main purpose is to protect brain cells
    b. It allows alcohol to pass directly to brain cells
    c. It does not allow some beneficial drugs to pass to brain cells
    d. It protects brain cells from nicotine and caffeine

17. All cells require ATP. ATP is the _____ of the cell.
    a. Protein manufacturer
    b. Transport center
    c. Energy currency
    d. Hereditary units

18. Which of the following are irregular bones?
    a. Facial and vertebrae
    b. Upper and lower limbs
    c. Skull and pelvis
    d. Wrists and ankles

19. The way the lower respiratory system is organized resembles, and is often referred to as, a bronchial _____.
    a. Root
    b. Leaf
    c. Tree
    d. Trunk

20. The causes of lymphedema can be:
    a. Congenital abnormality of lymphatic vessels
    b. Blockage to lymphatic vessels by a parasite
    c. Damage to lymphatic vessels following surgery
    d. All of the above

21. Which of the following statements regarding the urethra is true?
    a. It is shorter in women
    b. It transports both urine and semen in men
    c. It connects the bladder to the outside
    d. All of the above are true

22. Type 1 diabetes:
    a. Is not usually treated with insulin
    b. Is a disease of old age
    c. Is thought to be an autoimmune disease
    d. Can be treated with a low-protein diet

23. The sound created by the beating heart is due to the:
    a. Contraction of the ventricles
    b. Closing of the valves
    c. Movement of blood
    d. Contraction of the atria

24. Which of the following is not a skin infestation?
    a. Pediculosis corporis
    b. Tinea corporis
    c. Scabies
    d. Pediculosis capitis

25. The medulla oblongata:
    a. Regulates water balance and temperature balance
    b. Controls movement, posture, and balance
    c. Controls cardiac and respiratory centers
    d. Receives and processes sensory information

26. When an enzyme is _____ it can no longer function.
    a. Denatured
    b. Deaminated
    c. Detoxified
    d. Defecated

27. An example of an autoimmune disease is:
    a. Diabetes mellitus
    b. Rheumatoid arthritis
    c. Multiple sclerosis
    d. All of the above

28. External respiration occurs:
    a. In the lungs
    b. Between lungs and blood
    c. In cells
    d. Between blood and tissue cells

29. During walking, if the quadriceps are the prime movers then the _____ will be the antagonists.
    a. Gluteals
    b. Adductors
    c. Hamstrings
    d. Obliques

30. The secondary sex characteristics develop:
    a. At puberty in both boys and girls
    b. At the menarche in both boys and girls
    c. At the age of 11 in both boys and girls
    d. At the age of 14 in both boys and girls

31. The three bones that have fused together to form the innominate bone are:
    a. Ischium, pubis, ilium
    b. Ilium, sacrum, ischium
    c. Pelvis, sacrum, coccyx
    d. Pubis, sacrum, ilium

32. The adrenal glands are found:
    a. In the throat
    b. Above the kidneys
    c. In the abdomen
    d. Below the brain

33. The hepatic portal circulation involves the:
    a. Heart and the rest of the body
    b. Heart and the brain
    c. Heart and the lungs
    d. Heart and the digestive system

34. Starch, disaccharides, and lactose are all examples of:
    a. Proteins
    b. Enzymes
    c. Carbohydrates
    d. Lipids

35. A reflex action:
    a. Is under the control of the endocrine system
    b. Is under the control of the will
    c. Occurs without the involvement of the spinal cord
    d. Occurs without the involvement of the brain

36. Miliaria rubra (prickly heat) is a disorder of the:
    a. Sebaceous glands
    b. Nail bed
    c. Sweat glands
    d. Hair follicle

37. The cause of cystic fibrosis is:
    a. Genetic
    b. Viral
    c. Cancer
    d. Age

38. The soleus muscle lies _____ to the gastrocnemius muscle.
    a. Medial
    b. Deep
    c. Superficial
    d. Proximal

39. Which of these groups of lymph nodes is not found in the head and neck?
    a. Submandibular
    b. Axillary
    c. Occipital
    d. Parotid

40. The correct order of events in somatic cell division is:
    a. Metaphase, anaphase, telophase, prophase
    b. Telophase, prophase, anaphase, metaphase
    c. Prophase, metaphase, anaphase, telophase
    d. Anaphase, metaphase, telophase, prophase

41. Which of the following would indicate a "normal" range of blood pressure in a healthy person?
    a. Between 70 and 100 systolic and 20 and 50 diastolic
    b. Between 100 and 130 systolic and 60 and 90 diastolic
    c. Between 130 and 160 systolic and 90 and 120 diastolic
    d. Between 160 and 190 systolic and 120 and 150 diastolic

42. Hair loss can be caused by:
    a. Hormonal change
    b. Poor nutrition
    c. Emotional stress
    d. All of the above

43. In a cell-mediated response:
    a. Cells attack cells
    b. Cells attack antibodies
    c. Antibodies attack cells
    d. All of the above

44. Medication that can help women to cope with the effects of the menopause is:
    a. PID
    b. STD
    c. HRT
    d. PMT

45. The color of urine is determined by:
    a. Bile
    b. Blood
    c. Hormones
    d. Toxins

46. Pronation and supination refer to movements of the:
    a. Hands
    b. Knees
    c. Neck
    d. Abdomen

47. Hypersecretion from the adrenal cortex will not cause:
    a. Virilism
    b. Cushing's syndrome
    c. Diabetes insipidus
    d. Hirsutism

48. This part of the nail secures the nail to the finger or toe:
    a. Nail groove
    b. Nail plate
    c. Nail wall
    d. Nail bed

49. Each ureter drains the renal pelvis of a kidney and inserts into the _____ aspect of the bladder.
    a. Anterior
    b. Posterior
    c. Superior
    d. Inferior

50. Which of the following statements is false?
    a. Cutaneous membranes are found in joints
    b. Serous membranes do not open directly to the exterior
    c. Synovial membranes secrete synovial fluid
    d. A function of mucous membranes is protection

Practice Quiz 14

1. Which of the following glands produce oil to protect the skin and hair?
    a. Sebaceous
    b. Sweat
    c. Apocrine
    d. Eccrine

2. Light rays are received in the eye by photoreceptors on the _____.
    a. Aqueous humor
    b. Retina
    c. Vitreous humor
    d. Lens

3. Which of the following is not a function of the vertebral column?
    a. Supporting the head
    b. Protecting the spinal cord
    c. Allowing attachment for the ribs
    d. Protecting the heart and lungs

4. Infants are tested for adequate thyroid function at birth in order to prevent:
    a. Graves' disease
    b. Cretinism
    c. Goiter
    d. Cushing's disease

5. Which of the following is false regarding the pancreas?
    a. It is both an endocrine and an exocrine gland
    b. Many different enzymes are made and secreted by the pancreas
    c. Pancreatic juice is secreted from about a third of the pancreatic cells
    d. Pancreatic juice is of an alkaline nature

6. The function of the "stirrup" is to:
    a. Connect the middle ear with the upper portion of the throat
    b. Carry sound waves from the auricle to the eardrum
    c. Transmit sound waves to the inner ear
    d. Secrete cerumen

7. The inguinal lymph nodes are situated in the:
    a. Armpits
    b. Groin
    c. Abdomen
    d. Neck

8. Immunocompetent cells are:
    a. B cells
    b. T cells
    c. Both B and T cells
    d. Neither B nor T cells

9. Most of the respiratory passages are lined with:
   a. Ciliated epithelium
   b. Columnar epithelium
   c. Cuboid epithelium
   d. Cartilage

10. Which layer of the heart wall contracts to pump blood?
    a. Endocardium
    b. Pericardium
    c. Myocardium
    d. Epicardium

11. Reproductive cells are called:
    a. Gametes
    b. Meiosis
    c. Gonads
    d. Zygotes

12. The organ of Corti is found in the:
    a. Eye
    b. Tongue
    c. Ear
    d. Nose

13. An example of a condyloid joint can be found at the:
    a. Wrist
    b. Ankle
    c. Elbow
    d. Shoulder

14. Metastasis means:
    a. An allergic reaction to a metal
    b. The spread of cancer
    c. An infection of a lymph node
    d. The inability to destroy cancer cells

15. The iliopsoas muscle:
    a. Abducts the hip joint
    b. Extends the hip joint
    c. Adducts the hip joint
    d. Flexes the hip joint

16. Rennin is an enzyme found only in the stomachs of:
    a. Teenagers
    b. Women
    c. Infants
    d. Elderly people

17. Addison's disease is caused by:
    a. Hypersecretion from the thyroid gland
    b. Hypersecretion from the ovaries
    c. Hyposecretion from the adrenal cortex
    d. Hyposecretion from the parathyroids

18. Electrolytes in the blood are:
    a. Balanced by the kidneys
    b. Substances such as sodium, chloride, or potassium
    c. Affected by the water balance in the body
    d. All of the above

19. Macrophages within the alveoli are present in order to:
    a. Prevent infection
    b. Maximize oxygen uptake
    c. Prevent collapse
    d. Keep them moisturized

20. Which of the following is a false statement?
    a. Veins have a triple-layer wall just like arteries
    b. Veins have valves in their walls
    c. The lumen of a vein is usually smaller than that of an artery
    d. Veins usually carry blood toward the heart

21. This is a common bacterial infection, very contagious, and characterized by weeping yellow blisters or crusty sores:
    a. Impetigo
    b. Furuncle
    c. Hordeolum
    d. Boil

22. Vaccination is giving a _____ form of a disease to a person:
    a. High energy
    b. Artificial
    c. Weakened
    d. Inactive

23. Eccrine sweat glands do not produce:
    a. Urea
    b. Salts
    c. Hormones
    d. Water

24. The sensory receptors in the olfactory epithelium are:
    a. Gustatory receptors
    b. Photoreceptors
    c. Mechanoreceptors
    d. Chemoreceptors

25. Deoxygenated blood is brought to the lungs for gaseous exchange by the:
    a. Pulmonary veins
    b. Pulmonary arteries
    c. Bronchial arteries
    d. Bronchial veins

26. _____ is essential for muscle contraction.
    a. Carbon
    b. Nitrogen
    c. Calcium
    d. Hydrogen

27. Lipids arrive at the liver via:
    a. The hepatic artery
    b. The hepatic portal vein
    c. Both of the above
    d. Neither of the above

28. Movements at the feet can be:
    a. Inversion
    b. Dorsiflexion
    c. Plantarflexion
    d. All of the above

29. Which of the following is true?
    a. Passive immunity is when the body makes its own antibodies
    b. Vaccinations achieve immunity without recipients being ill
    c. Immunity lasts longer when ready-made antibodies are used
    d. Naturally acquired active immunity involves vaccination

30. "Blood pressure" is:
    a. The average amount of blood contained in the heart at any one time
    b. The force with which the valves are able to close
    c. The combined pressure of blood in the venous and capillary system
    d. The force exerted by the blood upon the walls of a blood vessel

31. An autoimmune disease affecting the myelin sheaths of nerves with periods of remission is likely to be:
    a. Myalgic encephalomyelitis
    b. Motor neurone disease
    c. Meningitis
    d. Multiple sclerosis

32. The innermost layer of the pleura is the _____ layer.
    a. Parietal
    b. Peripheral
    c. Visceral
    d. Varicose

33. Which of the following is a muscle of facial expression?
    a. Serratus anterior
    b. Risorius
    c. Temporalis
    d. Pterygoids

34. The temporomandibular joint is a _____ joint.
    a. Diarthrotic
    b. Synarthrotic
    c. Amphiarthrotic
    d. None of the above

35. The hypothalamus:
    a. Regulates posture and balance
    b. Coordinates sneezing and coughing
    c. Controls sensations of hunger and thirst
    d. Helps to control respiration

36. Nocturia may occur:
    a. At night
    b. In pregnant women
    c. Due to enlargement of the prostate gland
    d. All the above

37. Goblet cells in the digestive system secrete:
    a. Digestive juices
    b. Mucus
    c. Enzymes
    d. Saliva

38. The term "superficial" means:
    a. At the front of the body
    b. At the back of the body
    c. Toward the surface of the body
    d. Away from the surface of the body

39. At the capillary bed:
    a. Solutes from the blood pass into the interstitial fluid
    b. Pressure at the arteriolar end is higher than at the venous end
    c. Waste products can pass through the capillary wall because it is only one cell thick
    d. All of the above

40. A spasm could be defined as:
    a. An abnormal, involuntary muscular contraction
    b. A sudden painful contraction of a muscle
    c. Overstretching of a muscle
    d. Tearing of muscle fascia

41. Which of the following hormones is released by the anterior pituitary gland?
    a. Antidiuretic hormone (vasopressin)
    b. Thyroid-stimulating hormone
    c. Glucocorticoids
    d. All of the above

42. Which is the correct order of events regarding inspiration?
    a. Air is drawn into the lungs, the diaphragm contracts, the pressure in the thorax decreases, the volume in the thorax increases
    b. The volume in the thorax increases, air is drawn into the lungs, the pressure in the thorax decreases, the diaphragm contracts
    c. The diaphragm contracts, the volume in the thorax increases, the pressure in the thorax decreases, air is drawn into the lungs
    d. The pressure in the thorax decreases, the diaphragm contracts, air is drawn into the lungs, the volume in the thorax increases

43. A severe cramping pain in the lower back could be:
    a. Incontinence
    b. Renal colic
    c. Anuria
    d. Pyelitis

44. Cystitis commonly affects women because:
    a. Women have shorter ureters
    b. Women have weaker bladders
    c. Women have shorter urethras
    d. Women have smaller kidneys

45. The hormone(s) responsible for regulating the mineral content of the blood is(are):
    a. Glucagon
    b. Mineralocorticoids
    c. Glucocorticoids
    d. Thymosin

46. What is the function of areolar tissue?
    a. To surround body organs
    b. To move substances along a passageway

c. To line blood and lymphatic vessels

d. To allow organs to distend or expand

47. **Which of the following protects the nail bed from infection?**
    a. Cuticle
    b. Eponychium
    c. Hyponychium
    d. Nail wall

48. **An imaginary line that divides the body vertically into right and left portions is called the:**
    a. Sagittal plane
    b. Frontal plane
    c. Oblique plane
    d. Transverse plane

49. **The function of the vas deferens is to:**
    a. Store sperm until they are fully mature
    b. Transport sperm from the epididymis to the urethra
    c. Transport semen to the exterior of the body
    d. Produce sperm through the process of spermatogenesis

50. **A basic structured unit called a Haversian system is found in:**
    a. The alveoli
    b. A neuron
    c. Myofibrils
    d. Compact bone tissue

PART 3

Bringing It All Together

It is now your turn to have some fun and bring your knowledge of anatomy and physiology to life. So far, you have been studying **systemic** anatomy and physiology. Now, translate this knowledge into **regional** anatomy and physiology—in other words, take what you know and organize it into the regions of the body instead of the systems of the body.

On the following pages you will find the basic skeletal structure of a region. Draw and label the organs found in the region as well as the muscles, nerves, and lymphatic and blood vessels of the region. If you don't like drawing, then list them or do a spider diagram of them. It doesn't matter how you do it—as long as you know in your mind what goes where.

Then, next to each region jot down some notes on the most common diseases/disorders that affect that region. For example, common disorders of the head and neck are headaches, ear infections, and sinusitis. You should be able to list the causes, symptoms, and treatments of each of these disorders.

Skeletal Structure of the Head and Neck

Common diseases of the head and neck

Skeletal Structure of the Upper Limbs

Common diseases of the upper limbs

Skeletal Structure of the Back

Common diseases of the back

Skeletal Structure of the Chest

Common diseases of the chest

Skeletal Structure of the Abdomen

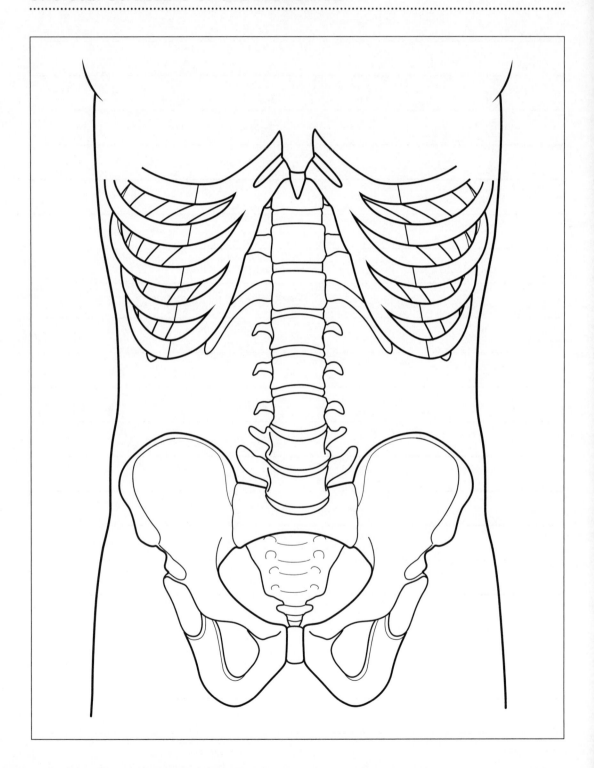

Common diseases of the abdomen

Skeletal Structure of the Pelvis

Common diseases of the pelvis

Skeletal Structure of the Lower Limbs

Common diseases of the lower limbs

Chronic Diseases

According to the World Health Organization, the most common chronic diseases are:

- Coronary artery disease (atherosclerosis)
- Cancer
- Stroke
- Asthma
- Type 2 diabetes mellitus.

It is important for you to have an in-depth understanding of how these diseases develop in the body and their signs and symptoms. Do some of your own research and complete the following table.

Disease	Coronary Artery Disease	Cancer	Stroke	Asthma	Type 2 Diabetes Mellitus
Risk factors					
Clinical signs					
Symptoms					
Medical treatment options					
Long-term effects (think about the effects on different systems of the body).					
Lifestyle recommendations					

Answer Key

Please note that no answers are provided for the review and self-study sections that form the first part of each chapter.

Chapter 1

Exercise 1

1. Lateral
2. Medial
3. Superior, cranial, or cephalad
4. Proximal
5. Distal
6. Superficial
7. Deep
8. Inferior or caudal
9. Midline or median line

Exercise 2

a. Superior
b. Inferior
c. Medial
d. Lateral
e. Proximal
f. Distal
g. Periphery

Exercise 3

1. h
2. d
3. b
4. g
5. c
6. j
7. a
8. e

9. i
10. f

Exercise 4

Dorsal cavity: brain, spinal cord
Thoracic cavity: esophagus, heart, lungs
Abdominal cavity: gall bladder, liver, pancreas
Pelvic cavity: urinary bladder, reproductive organs

Exercise 5

a. Sagittal plane
b. Frontal/coronal plane
c. Transverse plane
d. Oblique plane

Exercise 6

a. Chronic
b. Acute
c. Acute
d. Acute
e. Chronic
f. Chronic
g. Chronic
h. Acute
i. Acute
j. Acute

Exercise 7

a. Localized
b. Localized
c. Localized
d. Systemic
e. Systemic
f. Systemic
g. Localized
h. Systemic
i. Localized
j. Localized

Exercise 8

a. Sign
b. Sign
c. Symptom
d. Sign
e. Sign
f. Symptom
g. Sign
h. Sign
i. Symptom
j. Symptom

Exercise 9

a. Sympathetic
b. Fight-or-flight
c. Epinephrine (adrenaline)
d. Cortisol

Vocabulary test

a. The study of the structure of the body
b. Toward the head, above
c. Divides horizontally into inferior and superior portions
d. Farther from its origin or point of attachment of a limb
e. Line through the middle of the body
f. Relating to the inner walls of a body cavity
g. The study of the diseases of the body
h. The study of the functions of the body
i. At the front of the body, in front of
j. Relating to the internal organs of the body
k. Acute
l. Cachexia
m. Edema
n. Prognosis
o. Inflammation
p. Peripheral
q. Carpal
r. Chronic
s. Systemic
t. Etiology

Multiple-choice questions

1. c
2. a
3. b
4. d
5. b
6. d
7. a
8. c
9. a
10. b

Chapter 2

Plasma membrane

Generalized cell

Types of epithelial tissue cells

Structure of smooth muscle

Structure of cardiac muscle

Structure of skeletal muscle

Exercise 1

Across:
Magnesium
Calcium
Phosphorus
Nitrogen
Iodine
Chlorine

Down:
Hydrogen
Sodium
Iron
Oxygen
Carbon
Sulfur
Potassium

Exercise 2

a. Inorganic, water, temperature, lubricant, brain, solvent
b. Carbon, lipids, proteins, nucleic acids, adenosine triphosphate
c. Carbon, hydrogen, fuel/energy
d. Fats, carbon, hydrogen, oxygen
e. Carbon, hydrogen, oxygen, nitrogen, sulfur

Exercise 3

1. f
2. h
3. k
4. c
5. e
6. g
7. j
8. d
9. a
10. b
11. i

Exercise 4

a. Lysosome
b. Smooth endoplasmic reticulum
c. Nucleus
d. Site of protein synthesis
e. Barrier that surrounds the cell
f. Golgi body
g. Cytoplasm

Exercise 5

a. T
b. F
c. F
d. T
e. F
f. F
g. T
h. F
i. F
j. T

Exercise 6

a. Areolar tissue
b. Layers of cells that change shape to allow tissue to stretch
c. Intervertebral discs
d. Secretion and absorption
e. Ciliated simple columnar epithelium
f. Insulation, energy reserve, support, and protection
g. Elastic connective tissue/yellow elastic tissue
h. Heart wall
i. Mucous membranes
j. Lubrication and cushioning

Exercise 7

a. Lack of oxygen
b. Physical injury
c. Chemical injury
d. Infection
e. Immune-induced injury
f. Genetic defects
g. Nutritional imbalances

Exercise 8

Cancer

Exercise 9

Any four of the following are correct: surgery, radiation therapy, chemotherapy, immunotherapy, hormone therapy, targeted therapy.

Vocabulary test

a. The engulfment and destruction of microbes, cell debris, and foreign matter by phagocytes
b. A protein that speeds up the rate of a reaction without itself being used in the reaction
c. The process by which the body maintains a stable internal environment
d. Having two complete sets of chromosomes per cell
e. A small, fluid-filled sac
f. The changes that take place within the body to

enable its growth and function

g. Any cell except the reproductive cells

h. The basic unit of genetic material

i. A liquid in which a solid is dissolved

j. The energy of motion

k. Substance in the nucleus, made of DNA and proteins, that forms chromosomes during cellular replication

l. The removal of a sample of tissue for examination

m. A reduced or inadequate supply of blood to an area

n. The process by which the cell splits into new cells

o. The uncontrolled division of body cells

p. A reduced oxygen supply

q. Non-cancerous

r. The spread of cancer cells from their primary site to a secondary site

Multiple-choice questions

1. c
2. d
3. b
4. a
5. c
6. a
7. d
8. a
9. b
10. c
11. a
12. a
13. b
14. a
15. c

Chapter 3

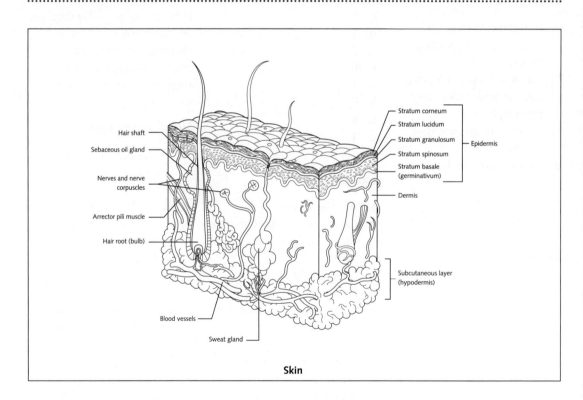

Hair shaft

Sebaceous oil gland

Nerves and nerve corpuscles

Arrector pili muscle

Hair root (bulb)

Blood vessels

Sweat gland

Stratum corneum

Stratum lucidum

Stratum granulosum

Stratum spinosum

Stratum basale (germinativum)

Epidermis

Dermis

Subcutaneous layer (hypodermis)

Skin

Hair

B: Nail

A: Finger cross-section

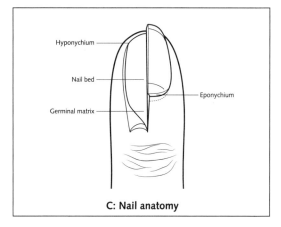

C: Nail anatomy

Exercise 1

b, d, e, f

Exercise 2

A. Asymmetry
B. Bleeding and border
C. Color
D. Diameter

Exercise 3

Any seven of the following: heat regulation, sensation, protection, absorption, excretion, secretion, vitamin D synthesis, immunity, blood reservoir, communication.

Exercise 4

a. Hair shaft
b. Sebaceous gland
c. Arrector pili muscle
d. Hair root
e. Hair follicle
f. Epidermis
g. Dermis
h. Subcutaneous tissue

Exercise 5

a. F
b. T
c. F
d. T
e. F

Exercise 6

1. d
2. f
3. b
4. g
5. c
6. h
7. a
8. e

Exercise 7

The correct order is d, b, e, a, c

Exercise 8

Across:
  3. Protection
  7. Root

9. Lanugo
12. Catagen
13. Eponychium
16. Telogen

Down:
1. Fold
2. Oil
3. Pili
4. Nostril
5. Shaft
6. Lunula
8. Terminal
10. Anagen
11. Papilla
14. Onyx
15. Bed

Exercise 9

a. Dermis, papillary, reticular
b. Papillary, areolar connective, elastic, papillae, capillaries
c. Reticular, dense irregular connective, collagen, elastic, hair, nerves, glands, sweat, adipose, reticular, subcutaneous, areolar connective, adipose

Exercise 10

a. Dry
b. Normal/balanced
c. Sensitive

Exercise 11

a. 2
b. 3
c. 2

d. 1
e. 1

Exercise 12

a. Eczema
b. Furuncle (boil)
c. Tinea capitis (scalp ringworm)
d. Tinea pedis (athlete's foot)
e. Chloasma
f. Vitiligo
g. Milia
h. Warts
i. Beau's lines
j. Paronychia
k. Tinea unguium (ringworm of the nail)

Exercise 13

1. c
2. f
3. h
4. n
5. a
6. p
7. l
8. q
9. o
10. k
11. e
12. m
13. g
14. i
15. d
16. j
17. b

Vocabulary test

a. Cross-infection
b. Desquamation
c. Integumentary system

d. Vasoconstriction
e. Vasodilation
f. An abnormal growth of tissue
g. The process through which cells die and become full of the protein keratin
h. The removal of the skin caused by scratching or scraping
i. A semi-solid or fluid-filled lump above and below the skin
j. The ingestion of bacteria by cells known as phagocytes
k. A crack in the skin that penetrates into the dermis
l. A common skin reaction in which there is swelling with redness and elevation
m. A thick, protective layer of skin caused by repeated pressure or friction

Multiple-choice questions

1. c
2. d
3. b
4. b
5. a
6. d
7. c
8. c
9. d
10. c
11. a
12. c
13. a
14. b
15. c

Chapter 4

Compact bone tissue

Spongy bone tissue

Structure of a long bone

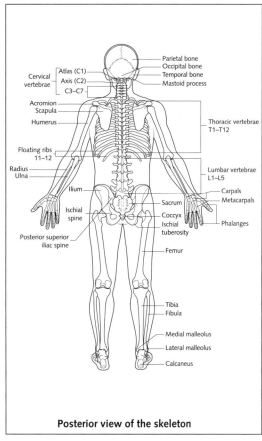

Posterior view of the skeleton

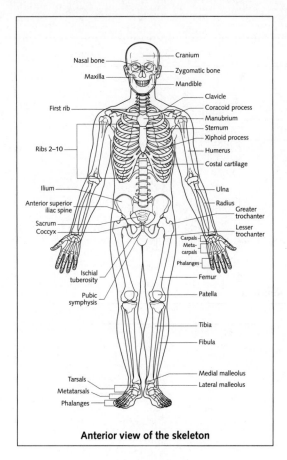

Anterior view of the skeleton

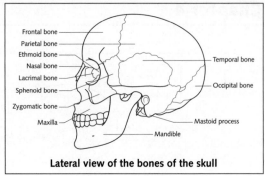

Lateral view of the bones of the skull

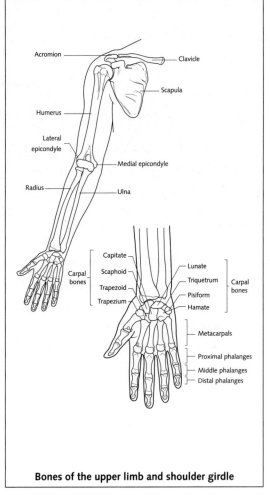

Bones of the upper limb and shoulder girdle

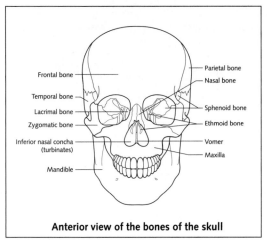

Anterior view of the bones of the skull

Lateral view of the pelvic girdle, lower limb, and foot

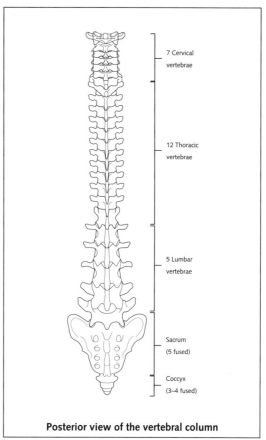

Posterior view of the vertebral column

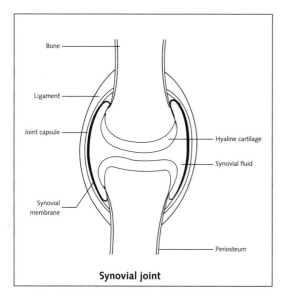

Synovial joint

Exercise 1

Across:
Energy storage
Hemopoiesis
Movement

Down:
Mineral homeostasis
Support
Protection

Exercise 2

a. Osteology, osseous, connective
b. Mineral, collagen, calcium, hydroxyapatite, hardness

Exercise 3

a. Compact (dense) bone tissue
b. Spongy (cancellous) bone tissue

Exercise 4

a. Long bone
b. Short bone
c. Flat bone
d. Irregular bone
e. Sesamoid bone

Exercise 5

1. d
2. f
3. b
4. g
5. c
6. a
7. e

Exercise 6

Axial, appendicular

Exercise 7

a. 7
b. 12
c. 5
d. 5
e. 4

Exercise 8

a. Hyoid
b. Sternum
c. Ribs

Exercise 9

Tarsals:
Talus
Medial cuneiform
Calcaneus
Navicular
Cuboid
Lateral cuneiform
Intermediate cuneiform

Carpals:
Scaphoid
Triquetrum
Pisiform
Hamate
Trapezoid
Lunate
Capitate
Trapezium

Exercise 10

a. F
b. T
c. F
d. T
e. T
f. F

Exercise 11

a. Flexing
b. Abducting
c. Supinating
d. Circumducting

Exercise 12

a. Condyloid (ellipsoid) joint
b. Hinge joint
c. Saddle joint
d. Pivot joint

e. Gliding (plane) joint
f. Ball-and-socket (spheroidal) joint

Exercise 13

a. Humerus, radius and ulna, carpal bones, metacarpal bones, proximal phalanges, middle phalanges, distal phalanges
b. Femur, patella, fibula and tibia, tarsal bones, metatarsal bones, proximal phalanges, middle phalanges, distal phalanges

Exercise 14

a, d

Exercise 15

a. Prolapsed intervertebral disc
b. Rheumatoid arthritis
c. Greenstick
d. Gout
e. Kyphosis
f. Osteoporosis
g. Lordosis
h. Hammer toes
i. Pes cavus
j. Scoliosis

Vocabulary test

a. A tough band of connective tissue that attaches muscles to bones
b. The process of bone formation

c. A tough band of connective tissue that attaches bones to bones

d. The production of blood cells and platelets

e. The point of contact between two bones—a joint

f. Air-filled space within the cranial and facial bones

g. The bones that are found in the center of the body (skull, hyoid, ribs, sternum, and vertebrae)

h. The central shaft of a long bone

i. Loss of calcium and other minerals from the bone matrix

j. Cells that destroy or resorb bone tissue

k. Pads of fibrocartilage found between the articular surfaces of bones; also called articular discs

l. An immovable joint

Multiple-choice questions

1. b
2. a
3. d
4. a
5. c
6. c
7. a
8. d
9. c
10. a
11. d
12. b
13. b
14. d
15. d

Chapter 5

Skeletal muscle tissue

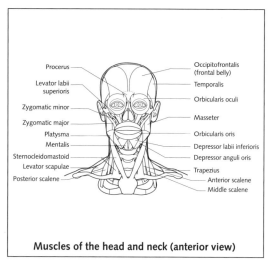

Muscles of the head and neck (anterior view)

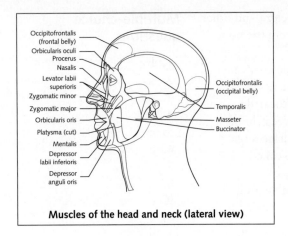

Occipitofrontalis (frontal belly)
Orbicularis oculi
Procerus
Nasalis
Levator labii superioris
Zygomatic minor
Zygomatic major
Orbicularis oris
Platysma (cut)
Mentalis
Depressor labii inferioris
Depressor anguli oris

Occipitofrontalis (occipital belly)
Temporalis
Masseter
Buccinator

Muscles of the head and neck (lateral view)

Occipitofrontalis (occipital belly)
Longissimus capitis
Trapezius

Muscles of the head and neck (posterior view)

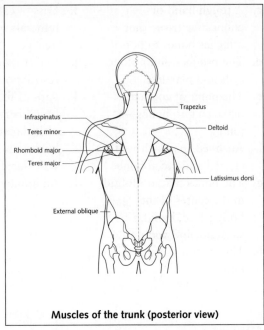

Infraspinatus
Teres minor
Rhomboid major
Teres major

Trapezius
Deltoid

External oblique

Latissimus dorsi

Muscles of the trunk (posterior view)

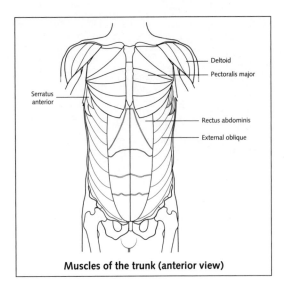

Serratus anterior

Deltoid
Pectoralis major

Rectus abdominis
External oblique

Muscles of the trunk (anterior view)

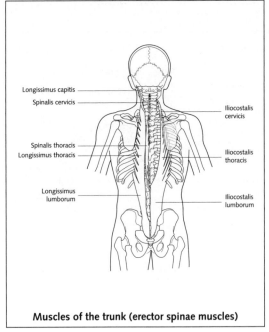

Longissimus capitis
Spinalis cervicis

Spinalis thoracis
Longissimus thoracis

Longissimus lumborum

Iliocostalis cervicis

Iliocostalis thoracis

Iliocostalis lumborum

Muscles of the trunk (erector spinae muscles)

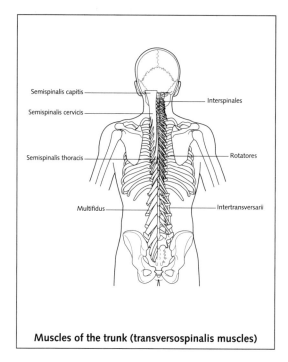

Muscles of the trunk (transversospinalis muscles)

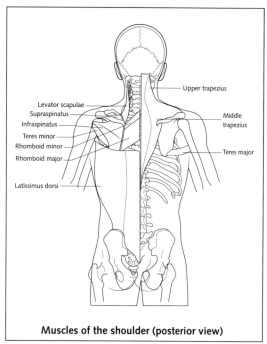

Muscles of the shoulder (posterior view)

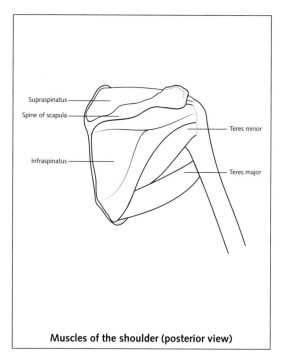

Muscles of the shoulder (posterior view)

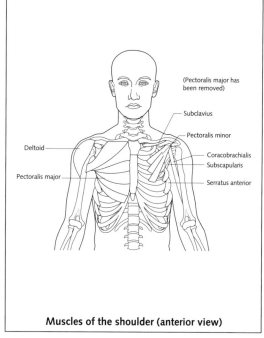

Muscles of the shoulder (anterior view)

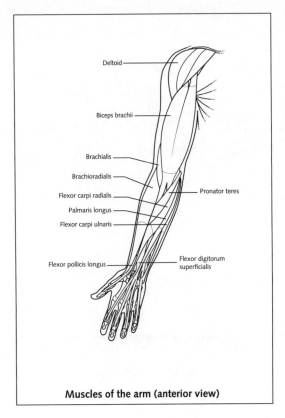

Muscles of the arm (anterior view)

Muscles of the leg (anterior view)

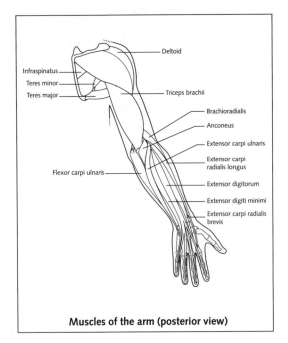

Muscles of the arm (posterior view)

Muscles of the leg (posterior view)

Exercise 1

Across:
3. ATP
4. Sarcomere
7. Epimysium
10. Glucose
11. Endomysium
14. Locomotion
16. Thermogenesis
17. Actin
18. Oxygen

Down:
1. Calcium
2. Tone
5. Fatigue
6. Visceral
8. Sarcolemma
9. Myofiber
12. Elasticity
13. Cardiac
15. Atony

Exercise 2

a. F
b. T
c. T
d. F
e. T
f. F
g. T
h. T
i. T
j. F

Exercise 3

a. Isotonic, isometric, isotonic, isometric
b. Isotonic, isometric
c. Oxygen

Exercise 4

a. White
b. Smallest
c. Walking and running

Exercise 5

a. 4
b. 3
c. 1
d. 5
e. 2

Exercise 6

a. Occipitalis
b. Orbicularis oculi
c. Orbicularis oris
d. Buccinator
e. Mentalis
f. Sternocleidomastoid

Exercise 7

Serratus anterior, rectus abdominis, pectoralis minor, pectoralis major

Exercise 8

Back:
Trapezius
Erector spinae
Latissimus dorsi

Arm:
Deltoid
Brachialis
Biceps brachii
Pronator teres
Supinator

Leg:
Gracilis
Sartorius
Soleus
Gastrocnemius
Tibialis anterior
Biceps femoris

Exercise 9

1. e
2. f
3. g
4. b
5. d
6. c
7. a

Exercise 10

a. Refer
b. Referral not necessary
c. Refer
d. Refer

Exercise 11

a. T
b. F
c. T
d. F
e. F
f. F

Vocabulary test

a. Aponeurosis
b. Atrophy
c. Fascia
d. Fibrosis
e. Hypertonia
f. Insertion

g. Origin
h. Tendon
i. Myositis
j. Spasm
k. Myalgia
l. Rheumatism
m. Glycolysis
n. Myopathy
o. Lumbago
p. Extensibility

Multiple-choice questions

1. b
2. b
3. a
4. d
5. d
6. a
7. c
8. d
9. b
10. d
11. c
12. a
13. d
14. c
15. b

Chapter 6

Motor neuron

Myelinated axon

Nerve

Ear

Brain

Mouth

Eye

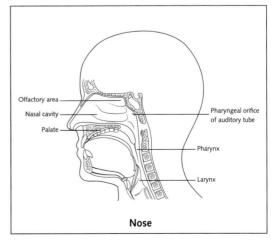

Nose

Exercise 1

Central nervous system (CNS):
The brain and spinal cord belong to the CNS. Its function is processing and integrating information.

Peripheral nervous system (PNS):
The cranial and spinal nerves belong to the PNS. Its function is carrying impulses.

Exercise 2

a. Somatic
b. Skeletal
c. Autonomic
d. Inhibits
e. Stimulates

Exercise 3

a. T
b. F
c. F
d. T
e. T
f. F

Exercise 4

a. Cell body
b. The receiving or input portion of a neuron
c. The transmitting portion of a neuron
d. Neurotransmitter
e. Synaptic vesicle
f. Sheath that protects and insulates neurons and speeds up the conduction of nerve impulses

g. Schwann cells (neurolemmocytes)
h. Gaps in the myelin sheath

Exercise 5

a. Diencephalon
b. Brain stem: midbrain, pons, medulla oblongata
c. Cerebrum
d. Cerebellum
e. Spinal cord

Exercise 6

a. Dura mater
b. Ventricles
c. Meninges
d. Arachnoid

Exercise 7

Across:
Limbic system
Cerebrum
Brain stem
Vagus
Abducens
Olfactory

Down:
Cerebellum
Diencephalon
Twelve
Cerebral cortex

Exercise 8

1. b
2. d
3. e
4. a
5. c

Exercise 9

a. 2
b. 4
c. 1
d. 3

Exercise 10

a. Outer/external, auricle/pinna, tympanic, vibrates, middle
b. Middle, eardrum/tympanic membrane, oval, round, hammer/malleus, anvil/incus, stirrup/stapes, auditory ossicles, Eustachian/auditory tube
c. Inner, perilymph, endolymph, vestibule, canals, Corti

Exercise 11

a. T
b. F
c. T
d. T
e. F

Exercise 12

a. Meningitis
b. Epilepsy
c. Anosmia
d. Alzheimer's disease
e. Spina bifida
f. Bell's palsy
g. Neuritis
h. Sciatica
i. Concussion
j. Glaucoma

Vocabulary test

a. Ganglion
b. Meninges
c. Neurology
d. Proprioceptor
e. Conductivity
f. Diencephalon
g. Cerebrospinal fluid
h. Ion
i. Irritability
j. Viscera

Multiple-choice questions

1. c
2. b
3. a
4. b
5. a
6. d
7. c
8. a
9. d
10. c
11. a
12. c
13. c
14. b
15. a

Chapter 7

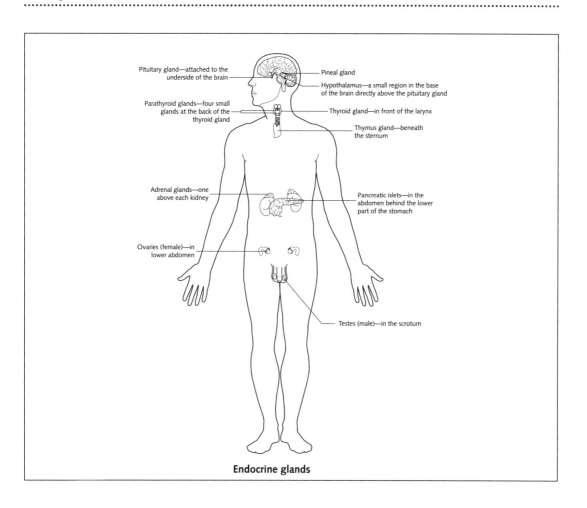

Endocrine glands

Exercise 1

a. F
b. T
c. F
d. T
e. F
f. F

Exercise 2

Pituitary:
Human growth hormone
Thyroid-stimulating hormone
Follicle-stimulating hormone
Luteinizing hormone
Prolactin
Adrenocorticotropic
 hormone
Melanocyte-stimulating
 hormone
Oxytocin
Antidiuretic hormone
 (vasopressin)

Pineal:
Melatonin

Thyroid:
Thyroid hormone
Calcitonin

Parathyroids:
Parathormone

Thymus:
Thymosin

Pancreas:
Glucagon
Insulin
Somatostatin

Adrenal cortex:
Mineralocorticoids
Glucocorticoids
Sex hormones

Adrenal medulla:
Epinephrine
Norepinephrine

Ovaries:
Estrogens
Progesterone

Testes:
Testosterone

Exercise 3

Across:
1. Pineal
3. Parathyroid
6. Hypothalamus
7. Exocrine
10. Testes
11. Hormone
13. Adrenal
14. Thyroid

Down:
1. Pituitary
2. Pancreas
4. Ovary
5. Endocrine
8. Reproduction
9. Medulla
12. Nervous
14. Thymus

Exercise 4

a. Hyposecretion
b. Diabetes mellitus
c. Calcium
d. Seasonal affective disorder
e. Acromegaly, gigantism
f. Antidiuretic (or
 vasopressin)
g. Goiter
h. Hypothyroidism
i. Graves'
j. Thyroid

Vocabulary test

a. The normal, ordered
 death and removal of cells
b. The study of the
 endocrine glands and the
 hormones they secrete
c. Sex organs that produce
 mature sex cells
d. Over- or excessive
 secretion
e. Under-secretion
f. Virilization
g. Goiter
h. Circadian rhythm
i. Catecholamines

Multiple-choice questions

1. b
2. a
3. d
4. a
5. b
6. c
7. c
8. d
9. b
10. a
11. c
12. a
13. c
14. b
15. d

Chapter 8

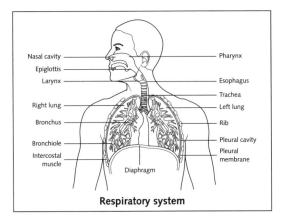

Respiratory system

Labels: Nasal cavity, Epiglottis, Larynx, Right lung, Bronchus, Bronchiole, Intercostal muscle, Diaphragm, Pharynx, Esophagus, Trachea, Left lung, Rib, Pleural cavity, Pleural membrane

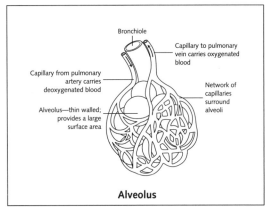

Alveolus

Labels: Bronchiole, Capillary to pulmonary vein carries oxygenated blood, Capillary from pulmonary artery carries deoxygenated blood, Network of capillaries surround alveoli, Alveolus—thin walled; provides a large surface area

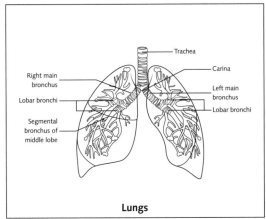

Lungs

Labels: Trachea, Right main bronchus, Lobar bronchi, Segmental bronchus of middle lobe, Carina, Left main bronchus, Lobar bronchi

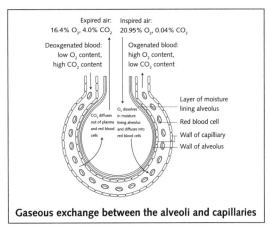

Gaseous exchange between the alveoli and capillaries

Labels: Expired air: 16.4% O_2, 4.0% CO_2; Inspired air: 20.95% O_2, 0.04% CO_2; Deoxgenated blood: low O_2 content, high CO_2 content; Oxgenated blood: high O_2 content, low CO_2 content; CO_2 diffuses out of plasma and red blood cells; O_2 dissolves in moisture lining alveolus and diffuses into red blood cells; Layer of moisture lining alveolus; Red blood cell; Wall of capilliary; Wall of alveolus

Exercise 1

1. d
2. a
3. e
4. f
5. g
6. c
7. b

Exercise 2

a. Nasal vestibule
b. Larynx
c. Right lung
d. Bronchus
e. Nasal cavity
f. Trachea
g. Left lung

Exercise 3

1. b and h
2. i and d
3. e
4. c
5. g
6. a
7. f

Exercise 4

a. Arteries, deoxygenated, oxygenated, veins
b. Bronchial, pulmonary, bronchial, vena cava

Exercise 5

a. T
b. F
c. T
d. T
e. F
f. F
g. T

Exercise 6

a. Asthma
b. Emphysema

c. Hyperventilation
d. Laryngitis
e. Rhinitis
f. Tuberculosis

7. k
8. i
9. a
10. l
11. b
12. f

4. c
5. d
6. a
7. c
8. b
9. a
10. d
11. d
12. b
13. c
14. a
15. a

Vocabulary test

1. g
2. e
3. d
4. h
5. j
6. c

Multiple-choice questions

1. a
2. c
3. b

Chapter 9

Heart

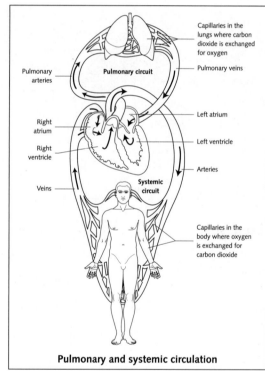

Pulmonary and systemic circulation

Exercise 1

Across:
3. Spleen
4. Solvent
6. Phagocytosis
8. Lymphocyte
9. Leucocyte
14. Electrolytes
15. Fibrinogen
17. Plasma

Down:
1. Waste
2. Hemoglobin
5. Basophil
7. Blood
10. Erythrocyte

11. Hemostasis
12. Neutrophil
13. Hormone
16. Oxygen

Exercise 2

a. Atrium, ventricle
b. Right, deoxygenated, lungs
c. Left, oxygenated, body
d. Backward, atrioventricular, semilunar

Exercise 3

a. Oxygenated
b. Heart
c. Heart
d. Heart tissue
e. Deoxygenated
f. Lungs
g. Most of the body superior to the diaphragm
h. Heart
i. Deoxygenated
j. Body inferior to the diaphragm
k. Deoxygenated
l. Oxygenated
m. Lungs

Exercise 4

a. Sinoatrial node
b. Systole
c. Cardiac cycle
d. Autorhythmic cells
e. Arterioles
f. Diastole

Exercise 5

a. Dave's blood pressure is high. Normal blood pressure is approximately 120/80 mm Hg.
b. The first figure, 160, is the systolic pressure and shows the pressure of the blood during contraction. The second figure, 100, is the diastolic pressure and shows the pressure of the blood during relaxation.

Exercise 6

1. b
2. f
3. c
4. a
5. e
6. d
7. g
8. h

Exercise 7

a. F
b. T
c. F
d. F
e. T
f. T
g. F
h. F
i. T
j. F

Exercise 8

a. Sepsis
b. Stroke

c. Shock
d. Heart attack

Exercise 9

a. Myocardial infarction
b. Bradycardia
c. Hemorrhoids
d. Epistaxis
e. Thrombus
f. Hypertension

Exercise 10

a. Relaxation of the heart muscle during the cardiac cycle
b. Contraction of the heart muscle during the cardiac cycle
c. The constriction of blood vessels
d. The dilation of blood vessels

Multiple-choice questions

1. b
2. a
3. c
4. a
5. d
6. d
7. a
8. a
9. d
10. c
11. b
12. a
13. d
14. d
15. c

Chapter 10

Lymph node

Lymphatic organs

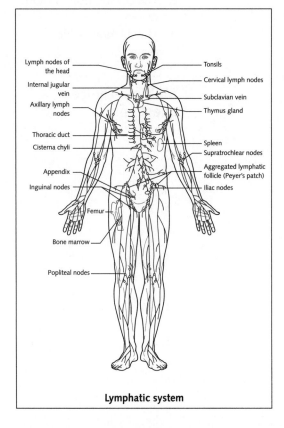

Lymphatic system

Exercise 1

a. Drains interstitial fluid
b. Transports dietary lipids
c. Protects against invasion

Exercise 2

a. F
b. T
c. T
d. F
e. T

Exercise 3

a. 4
b. 3
c. 1
d. 2

Exercise 4

Across:
Supratrochlear
Superficial parotid
Mastoid
Ileocolic
Cervical
Inguinal

Down:
Submandibular
Submental
Axillary
Occipital
Iliac
Popliteal

Exercise 5

Non-specific resistance to disease:
Mechanical barriers, natural killer cells, fever, chemical barriers, phagocytes, inflammation

The immune response:
T cells, B cells, immunological memory

Exercise 6

a. Lymphedema
b. Leukemia
c. Hodgkin's disease
d. Acquired immunodeficiency syndrome (AIDS)
e. Glandular fever

Exercise 7

1. f
2. g
3. e
4. a
5. b
6. c
7. d

Vocabulary test

a. A specialized protein that is synthesized to destroy a specific antigen
b. Any substance that the body recognizes as foreign
c. A scavenger cell that engulfs and destroys microbes
d. The spread of disease from its site of origin
e. A cell that is able to engulf and digest microbes

Multiple-choice questions

1. b
2. c
3. a
4. b
5. d
6. a
7. b
8. c
9. d
10. d
11. a
12. d
13. c
14. d
15. b

Chapter 11

Digestive system

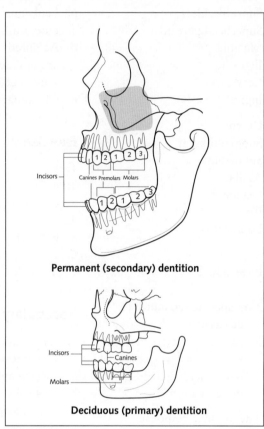

Permanent (secondary) dentition

Deciduous (primary) dentition

Exercise 1

Across:
4. Cecum
5. Chyme
6. Mastication
8. Colon
10. Defecation
12. Mouth
13. Parotid
16. Lipases
17. Bile
18. Alimentary canal
20. Dentes
21. Bolus

Down:
1. Anus
2. Deglutition
3. Amylase
7. Duodenum
9. Peritoneum
11. Ingestion
12. Monosaccharides
13. Peristalsis
14. Liver
15. Esophagus
19. Mucosa

Exercise 2

Mouth:
Salivary amylase
Lingual lipase

Stomach:
Gastric lipase
Pepsin
Rennin

Small intestine:
Pancreatic amylase
Trypsin
Pancreatic lipase
Bile

Intestinal juice
Brush border enzymes

Large intestine:
Bacteria

Exercise 3

a. T
b. F
c. F
d. T
e. F

Exercise 4

1. g. Mouth
2. h. Esophagus
3. a. Stomach
4. f. Pancreas
5. b. Small intestine
6. e. Large intestine
7. c. Gall bladder
8. d. Liver

Exercise 5

1. c
2. h
3. b
4. f
5. a
6. j
7. d

8. e
9. g
10. i

Exercise 6

a, d, e, f, i

Vocabulary test

a. The uptake of digested nutrients into the bloodstream and lymphatic system
b. A substance that alters the rate of a chemical reaction without itself being changed by the reaction
c. The process by which large molecules of food are broken down into smaller molecules that can enter cells
d. The substance on which an enzyme acts
e. Yellowing of the skin or whites of eyes due to high levels of bilirubin
f. Process by which indigestible substances are eliminated from the body
g. Bad breath

h. Excessive accumulation of interstitial fluid in body tissues
i. Process of swallowing
j. Process of chewing food

Multiple-choice questions

1. b
2. d
3. a
4. c
5. a
6. b
7. c
8. c
9. d
10. a
11. b
12. d
13. b
14. c
15. b

Chapter 12

Kidney

Urinary system

Exercise 1

1. f
2. d
3. e
4. a
5. b
6. c

Exercise 2

a. Blood, urine
b. Adrenal/suprarenal
c. Cortex, medulla, pelvis
d. Nephrons

Exercise 3

a, f, d, h, g, i, e, b, c

Exercise 4

a. Afferent arteriole
b. Efferent arteriole
c. Proximal convoluted tubule
d. Distal convoluted tubule
e. Collecting duct
f. Medullary loop (loop of Henle)
g. Glomerular capsule
h. Glomerulus
i. Branch of renal vein
j. Branch of renal artery

Exercise 5

From the list, the following should be crossed out: hemoglobin, pus, glucose, proteins, red blood cells, bile pigments.

Exercise 6

a. T
b. F
c. T
d. F
e. T

Exercise 7

1. e
2. a
3. d
4. b
5. c

Vocabulary test

1. Polyuria
2. Dysuria
3. Proteinuria
4. Hematuria
5. Anuria
6. Oliguria
7. Nocturia

Multiple-choice questions

1. b
2. a
3. c
4. d
5. b
6. a
7. c
8. d
9. b
10. a
11. c
12. b
13. a
14. c
15. b

Chapter 13

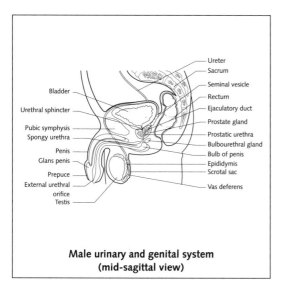

Male urinary and genital system (mid-sagittal view)

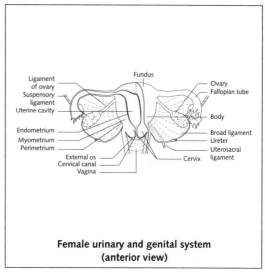

Female urinary and genital system (anterior view)

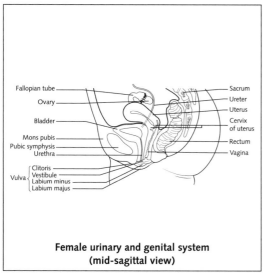

Female urinary and genital system (mid-sagittal view)

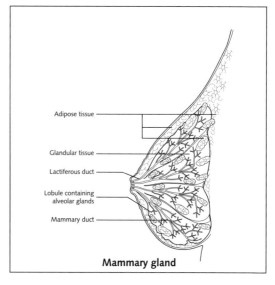

Mammary gland

Exercise 1

a. Meiosis is reproductive cell division in which four daughter cells are produced, each one having only 23 chromosomes, and it results in sperm and egg cells being produced. Together these cells can form a new organism.

b. Mitosis is somatic cell division and it occurs when the body needs to replace dead and injured cells or produce new cells for growth. It is the process in which a single diploid parent cell duplicates itself to produce two identical daughter cells.

Exercise 2

a. 4
b. 2
c. No
d. Yes
e. 23
f. 46

Exercise 3

Male:
Scrotum, penis, testes, epididymis, bulbourethral glands, spermatic cord, prostate, seminal vesicles, vas deferens

Female:
Ovaries, vulva, vagina, fallopian tubes, mammary glands, uterus

Exercise 4

a. F
b. T
c. F
d. F
e. T

Exercise 5

a. Menstruation
b. Oocyte
c. Fallopian tubes
d. Endometrium
e. Corpus luteum
f. Graafian follicle

Exercise 6

The correct description is **b.**

Exercise 7

a. Prostatitis
b. Ectopic pregnancy
c. Mastitis
d. Amenorrhea
e. Polycystic ovary syndrome (Stein-Leventhal syndrome)

Exercise 8

c and **g** should be circled.

Exercise 9

1. e
2. g
3. f
4. a
5. d
6. b
7. c

Vocabulary test

a. Fertilization
b. Haploid cell
c. Lactation
d. Oogenesis
e. Semen (seminal fluid)

Multiple-choice questions

1. b
2. c
3. d
4. a
5. c
6. d
7. d
8. c
9. b
10. a
11. d
12. c
13. a
14. b
15. b

Practice Quizzes

Quiz 1
1. a
2. b
3. d
4. b
5. d
6. c
7. c
8. d
9. c
10. b
11. c
12. b
13. a
14. c
15. a
16. b
17. b
18. a
19. d
20. a
21. d
22. c
23. a
24. c
25. d

Quiz 2
1. b
2. c
3. b
4. a
5. b
6. c
7. d
8. d
9. b
10. d
11. a
12. b
13. b
14. a
15. d
16. c
17. a
18. c
19. c
20. c
21. b
22. a
23. d
24. c
25. c

Quiz 3
1. d
2. b
3. a
4. c
5. b
6. d
7. b
8. a
9. c
10. d
11. b
12. a
13. d
14. c
15. c
16. b
17. a
18. b
19. c
20. b
21. b
22. a
23. d
24. a
25. d

Quiz 4
1. c
2. b
3. a
4. c
5. b
6. c
7. b
8. a
9. a
10. d
11. b
12. b
13. a
14. d
15. c
16. c
17. d
18. a
19. c
20. a
21. c
22. b
23. a
24. b
25. d

Quiz 5
1. c
2. d
3. c
4. b
5. d
6. c
7. b
8. c
9. d
10. b
11. a
12. c
13. c
14. d
15. c
16. d
17. b
18. c
19. b
20. a
21. c
22. d
23. d
24. b
25. c
26. d
27. c
28. a
29. b
30. c
31. c
32. a
33. a
34. d
35. b
36. d
37. c
38. c
39. a
40. b
41. c
42. c
43. d
44. b
45. b
46. d
47. b
48. c
49. a
50. b

Quiz 6
1. d
2. a
3. d
4. c
5. c
6. d
7. c
8. a
9. a
10. b
11. d
12. c
13. c
14. b
15. d
16. b
17. a
18. d
19. b
20. c
21. d
22. c
23. a
24. b
25. b
26. d
27. c
28. d
29. d
30. a
31. b
32. d
33. c
34. a
35. a
36. c
37. b
38. c
39. a
40. d
41. d
42. d
43. c
44. c
45. c
46. b
47. c
48. a
49. d
50. d

Quiz 7
1. c
2. a
3. b
4. a
5. d
6. c
7. d
8. b
9. d
10. d
11. c
12. a
13. c
14. d
15. c
16. a
17. c
18. d
19. c
20. c
21. c
22. b
23. d
24. b
25. c
26. d
27. b
28. d
29. c
30. d
31. b
32. b
33. d
34. d
35. a
36. c
37. a
38. b
39. c
40. d
41. a
42. c
43. b
44. d
45. d
46. a
47. d
48. c
49. b
50. d

Quiz 8
1. b
2. a
3. c
4. a
5. b
6. a
7. b
8. d
9. d
10. c
11. b
12. b
13. d
14. c
15. b
16. c
17. d
18. a
19. d
20. a
21. a
22. d
23. a
24. b
25. a
26. b
27. d
28. b
29. a
30. b
31. c
32. c
33. a
34. b
35. d
36. d
37. b
38. a
39. b
40. c
41. a
42. b
43. c
44. c
45. b
46. c
47. b
48. b
49. c
50. b

Quiz 9
1. a
2. b
3. c
4. a

5. d
6. c
7. d
8. a
9. c
10. b
11. d
12. b
13. c
14. d
15. d
16. b
17. a
18. c
19. b
20. c
21. b
22. b
23. a
24. d
25. d
26. b
27. c
28. b
29. a
30. b
31. a
32. c
33. d
34. d
35. a
36. c
37. b
38. b
39. a
40. d
41. c
42. d
43. a
44. b
45. c

46. d
47. a
48. d
49. b
50. c

Quiz 10

1. d
2. b
3. d
4. c
5. b
6. a
7. c
8. b
9. d
10. d
11. a
12. b
13. d
14. d
15. a
16. c
17. b
18. b
19. c
20. a
21. b
22. c
23. a
24. b
25. a
26. b
27. c
28. d
29. b
30. c
31. a
32. c
33. a

34. b
35. c
36. c
37. d
38. c
39. b
40. c
41. c
42. b
43. d
44. d
45. a
46. b
47. a
48. d
49. c
50. a

Quiz 11

1. d
2. a
3. a
4. c
5. b
6. b
7. c
8. b
9. d
10. d
11. c
12. b
13. d
14. b
15. a
16. d
17. d
18. c
19. d
20. b
21. a

22. c
23. a
24. c
25. d
26. a
27. a
28. c
29. b
30. d
31. b
32. c
33. b
34. a
35. d
36. b
37. b
38. d
39. c
40. b
41. a
42. d
43. b
44. d
45. a
46. a
47. c
48. b
49. d
50. a

Quiz 12

1. d
2. c
3. a
4. a
5. b
6. b
7. c
8. b
9. d

10. b
11. a
12. d
13. b
14. c
15. d
16. a
17. a
18. b
19. c
20. b
21. c
22. a
23. b
24. d
25. b
26. b
27. a
28. d
29. d
30. c
31. d
32. a
33. c
34. b
35. d
36. c
37. b
38. d
39. b
40. a
41. c
42. c
43. a
44. d
45. d
46. a
47. c
48. d
49. b
50. c

Quiz 13

1. a
2. b
3. c
4. a
5. c
6. c
7. d
8. c
9. b
10. a
11. c
12. b
13. c
14. d
15. a
16. d
17. c
18. a
19. c
20. d
21. d
22. c
23. b
24. b
25. c
26. a
27. d
28. b
29. c
30. a
31. a
32. b
33. d
34. c
35. d
36. c
37. a
38. b
39. b

40. c
41. b
42. d
43. a
44. c
45. a
46. a
47. c
48. d
49. b
50. a

Quiz 14

1. a
2. b
3. d
4. b
5. c
6. c
7. b
8. c
9. a
10. c
11. a
12. c
13. a
14. b
15. d
16. c
17. c
18. d
19. a
20. c
21. a
22. c
23. c
24. d
25. b
26. c
27. a

28. d
29. b
30. d
31. d
32. c
33. b
34. a
35. c
36. b
37. b
38. c
39. d
40. a
41. b
42. c
43. b
44. c
45. b
46. a
47. c
48. a
49. b
50. d